WRESTLING FOR TRUTH

WRESTLING FOR TRUTH

ONE MAN'S SEARCH FOR HEALTH, FAMILY, AND THE IDEAL LIFE

BLAKE SHUMATE

Advantage | Books

Published by Advantage Books, Charleston, South Carolina.
An imprint of Advantage Media.

Printed in the United States of America.

10 9 8 7 6 5 4 3 2 1

ISBN: 978-1-64225-907-0 (Paperback)
ISBN: 978-1-64225-906-3 (eBook)

Library of Congress Control Number: 2025915388

Cover design by Lance Buckley.
Layout design by Ruthie Wood.

Advantage Books is an imprint of Advantage Media Group. Advantage Media helps busy entrepreneurs, CEOs, and leaders write and publish a book to grow their business and become the authority in their field. Advantage authors comprise an exclusive community of industry professionals, idea-makers, and thought leaders. For more information go to **advantagemedia.com**.

08-26-2025 12:36

CONTENTS

DISCLAIMER

This is a memoir based on the author's personal experiences, memories, and reflections. The events described are true to the best of the author's recollection. The narrative represents the author's perspective and is not intended as a comprehensive or objective account of the events or individuals involved.

To protect privacy, some names and identifying details have been changed or altered. Certain characters may be composites or fictionalized representations of real people. Any resemblance to actual persons, living or dead, outside the context of the author's lived experience, is purely coincidental.

The intent of this work is to share a journey of growth, faith, and resilience. It is not intended to defame, harm, or misrepresent any individual, organization, or group.

FOREWORD

Life is full of challenges that test not just our strength but also our ability to adapt, grow, and find purpose in the face of adversity. For Blake Shumate, the journey of living with multiple sclerosis (MS) has been one such test—a deeply personal and transformative experience that reshaped his understanding of what it means to live a meaningful life.

In his book, Blake shares a powerful story of perseverance, reflection, and faith. But this isn't just a story of survival; it's a story of thriving, of finding purpose and clarity, even in the midst of profound uncertainty. As I read Blake's journey, I couldn't help but see the profound alignment between his mindset and the framework we use at The Ideal Life, which we call the I GOT This framework.

At its core, the I GOT This framework is about cultivating a growth mindset—a belief that challenges are not insurmountable obstacles but opportunities to grow, learn, and become more deliberate in the way we live. Blake's story is a living testament to this mindset. Through his struggles with MS, he has not only come to understand his own purpose on a deeper level but has also embraced the hard, deliberate work of building a life centered on what truly matters.

Blake's mindset is one of resilience and intentionality. As he faced the physical and emotional challenges that MS brought into his life, he didn't retreat or give up. Instead, he leaned into the struggle, using it as a catalyst for self-reflection and growth. He turned to his faith in God for guidance, grounding himself in spiritual truths that provided strength and perspective. He also became deeply intentional about nurturing his relationships with family, recognizing that these connections were a source of both purpose and joy.

What stands out most about Blake's approach, however, is how practical it is. This is not a book filled with abstract ideas or lofty philosophies—although both philosophy and faith have played a crucial role in his journey. Instead, Blake shares specific, actionable steps he has taken to fight back against MS, to reclaim control over his life, and to focus on what he can do rather than what he cannot. This mirrors one of the key principles of the I GOT This framework: the idea that growth comes from consistent, intentional action.

In my work at The Ideal Life, I've seen firsthand how transformative this kind of mindset can be. It's one thing to believe in the power of growth and purpose; it's another to live it out day by day, through deliberate choices and actions. Blake's story is an inspiring example of what it looks like to do just that. His journey reminds us that even when we face challenges that feel overwhelming, there are always things within our control—things we can do to move forward, to grow, and to live a life aligned with our values and purpose.

Another key principle of the I GOT This framework is the importance of having a coach or guide—someone who can offer perspective, encouragement, and practical advice. Blake's book serves as just that: a guide for anyone who is navigating their own challenges, whether they are living with MS or facing other obstacles in life. Blake doesn't just share his story; he offers insights and strategies that readers can apply to their own lives. In doing so, he becomes a kind of coach, walking alongside his readers and helping them see that they, too, can find strength, purpose, and growth in the face of adversity.

What makes Blake's journey particularly compelling is the way it combines faith and practicality. His deep trust in God has been a source of strength and guidance, helping him see the bigger picture and focus on what truly matters. At the same time, he has embraced the practical work of living with intention—taking deliberate steps to care for his body, nurture his relationships, and live in alignment with his values. This combination of faith and action is a powerful model for anyone seeking to live a purposeful life.

As you read this book, I encourage you to reflect on your own journey. What challenges are you facing right now? How might you approach them with the same mindset Blake has cultivated—a mindset that sees challenges as opportunities, that focuses on what is within your control, and that stays grounded in a sense of purpose?

Blake's story reminds us that the journey to a purposeful life isn't about achieving perfection or avoiding hardship. It's about showing up, day after day, with a commitment to growth, a reliance on faith, and a determination to focus on what truly matters. It's about doing the work, even when it's hard, and trusting that the effort will be worth it.

It's not a quick fix or an easy answer; it's a way of thinking and living that helps us move forward, even when the road is difficult. Blake's story is a powerful example of what this mindset looks like in action, and his book is a gift to anyone who is ready to embrace their own challenges as opportunities for growth.

As you turn the pages of this book, let Blake's story inspire you. Let it remind you that no matter what you are facing, you have the strength to grow, the ability to take action, and the capacity to find purpose in the midst of difficulty. And let it encourage you to take the next step on your own journey—knowing that, with the right mindset and the right guidance, you, too, can say, "I GOT This."

Mark Congdon
Founder and CEO of The Ideal Life

If you know me, then you know this isn't about me …

CHAPTER ONE
MY LIFE BEFORE

If I force myself to think about it, my life growing up—those years before I became who I am today—there isn't much emotion in the memories. The remembrances come slowly at first. They're light before they get heavy. Then they give way like a trap door with too much weight on it. The memories flood my mind, as unsettling as they are gratifying, and I'm left searching for words. But those memories are relieving to me. They're relieving because I still have them at all.

It's different for everyone, but some of the areas that multiple sclerosis (MS) may begin to affect are your brain's memory functions, along with mobility, stamina, flexibility, appetite, mood stabilization, and a host of other capabilities that we often take for granted. I decided to write this book to relay, as best I can, some of the gratitude I now feel for my life before MS—but also to explore the recognition and appreciation I have today living with MS. I choose to see this part of my life as a blessing. This is an opportunity to surrender control to my Lord and Savior, Jesus (Yeshua) Christ. He accepts and loves me despite my flaws. Through this reflection, He is motivating me to live more like He did by simply focusing on one thing: love. Perhaps the single most important thing we can find in ourselves and in others is the willingness to give love as easily as we accept it.

For me, the story of family begins with an act of both hopeful optimism and defiance.

When the doctors told my parents that after having me, they would likely never have another healthy child, they didn't believe them. Or at least they didn't *want* to believe them, so they decided to try for a second child anyway. My sister, Crystal Nicole, was born three years later with a condition doctors and specialists called "moderate mental retardation." It means that her IQ was somewhere between a score of thirty-five and forty-nine, well below the lowest percentile that is usually considered by schools, major corporations, government agencies, and other institutions that review such tests.

The condition rendered her unable to speak intelligibly, though she and I eventually learned to understand one another. We had no other choice. After my parents divorced when I was six, I became something of an adult myself. It was my responsibility to look after Crystal. I was to comfort her when she was scared or upset, to help feed her, to be simultaneously her big brother and her caregiver in the absence of our mother, who lived with us but worked twelve-hour shifts at a nearby textile factory.

Here's a memory: I don't ever remember feeling more than a certain numbness when the final school bell rang. From as early as I can recall, I felt that I was on my own. I would walk to the bus, watching the other kids getting into their parents' cars or talking excitedly with their friends as they boarded the bus. I got along with nearly everyone, but I didn't have many close friends. I rarely felt the way I assumed my peers were feeling as I watched them run to their parents' cars after school or jumped around together after a sporting event or some other kind of social gathering. One day, though, I was excited. I was excited because I knew that my Uncle Mike, a youth pastor and Crystal's best friend, was taking over the duty of caring for Crystal from Poppa Ralph, my mother's father, which didn't occur very often.

Uncle Mike was the kind of person who, if you ever saw him, you saw him smiling. He was kind and gentle, with a disarming and joyful presence that he carried wherever he went. Uncle Mike understood Crystal as well as I did. He conversed with her, showed her pictures, and read her passages from the Bible or other books. I knew she would be even happier than usual when I arrived home that day.

I settled into my seat, my bookbag in my lap. As we drove along the winding rural roads of Martinsville, Virginia, I gazed out of the bus window and began to think about everything I must do in order to go out on a bike ride later that evening. I learned at a very young age that cleaning up and keeping things in order made everything much easier to manage. I would think through each room, imagine the way it should be in order to meet my mother's satisfaction, and then decide where and how I should entertain Crystal while I worked to meet those specifications. When I got home, I would simply make those thoughts come to life. I knew that if everything was perfect around the house and Crystal was in a good mood, I would be able to head out on an adventure when Mom got home.

When we arrived at my stop, I got off the bus and took my usual shortcuts through the fields and backyards for a few blocks to my house. As I walked through the front door, I saw my sister's face, her eyes wide and her mouth agape, hands clapping. Uncle Mike came when he could, but Crystal was usually taken care of by my grandfather. Poppa was a good man, the kind of person who everyone needed, and he always obliged himself to help. On days when Crystal was going to get home before me, Poppa would come over to look after her until I got there. Sometimes, I would make Crystal and myself snacks and entertain her with games or simply set up some activity that would hold her attention. Crystal loved puzzles and could put them together upside down solely by looking at the shapes as opposed to the picture on the box. She also loved to be outside. If it was even close to being warm enough, she wanted to be in the aboveground pool in our backyard.

Even though Crystal was mentally handicapped, she brought a lot of joy to my life. She was much smarter than anyone seemed to think she was. I saw examples of it every day—from her understanding my humor to her thwarting my mother's and my attempts to prevent her from sneaking Oatmeal Creme Pies from the top of the cupboard. I learned to control her environment to keep her both safe and entertained, and she learned to understand the meaning of my words and the tools I used to control that environment—something I felt she needed. To this day, I struggle with understanding people's choices of words they use to communicate, but I'm skilled at reading people's behaviors in order to determine how things are defined within their paradigm. I believe I have Crystal to thank for that ability, as well as for my willingness to direct others and stand up for people who can't stand up for themselves. Without her, I don't believe I would have developed those skills, which are now invaluable in my life.

My mother, Tammy, on the other hand, felt cold and distant to me at the time, and we rarely exchanged more than a few words. She normally returned home from work between seven and eight o'clock in the evening. She was strict, going so far as to count snacks, drinks, and other items in the kitchen and scolding me if Crystal or I had eaten more of something than she felt we should have. Mom could remember everything. She was always quick to point out where a chair had been moved a few inches or a coaster had been left out of place and other things of little consequence to most people.

She rarely said very much to me, hardly any thank-yous, pats on the back, or inquiries into how my day was or what was happening at school. My memories of her in the evenings back then rarely extend beyond motorcycles, boyfriends, or country music. Mostly, I would see her sitting quietly, staring at the TV. I remember looking down the hall and seeing her sitting on the couch with her arms crossed, one leg over the other, the top leg steadily rocking. She would loosely squeeze a Marlboro Light cigarette in her hand, a stream of gray smoke streaking toward the ceiling above her head. If I ever did come out and sit with her in the living room, there would be no conversation, not a single word. It was as though she were away in some far-off place and only her body was present. I felt more comfortable either staying in my room or not being there at all.

I learned early to present myself as an adult to maintain the silence to which I had grown accustomed. Once home, I would wait for the silence. Hearing no complaints, I understood this to be good news. I would jump on my bike and ride off into the night. In my mind, I had finished my shift just as she had finished hers, so I could clock out, and we could stay out of each other's way.

I had two close friends who lived within biking distance from me: Robert and Solomon. We were typical school-aged boys, and as such, we played basketball and tennis, raced our bicycles, wrestled one another, and explored in the woods. I never had to be home at any specific time, so I was the kid who never wanted to go home and always wanted their friends to break curfew. Robert was my go-to friend to stay out later with, as he had a two-story condo, a bedroom window that accessed his roof, and a walk-out basement perfect for late-night escape routes. He could climb out, or I could go in through the basement without his parents knowing, and we would sit around talking as late as we wanted to. But, of course, most of the other neighborhood kids had to go home early, at least in my eyes. Then, one afternoon when I was in the fourth grade, I met two new kids who would alter the course of my young life.

I still remember that after-school bus ride vividly. I was seated toward the middle of the bus when I heard a commotion coming from the rear. When I turned to see what was happening, I saw a group of my classmates teasing a heavyset boy whom I didn't recognize. Next to him was a younger boy who looked about as big as a dot in an exclamation point. The larger boy sat calmly, ignoring everyone and staring straight ahead, while the small one stood up in his seat and began yelling back at the group of kids bullying the boy whom I learned later was his brother. I, too, stood up and told the other kids to stop teasing them. Before I knew what was happening, this little dot began aiming his exclamation point at me. "We can take care of ourselves! You sit down and stay out of it!" he shouted. Confused and stunned, I returned to my seat and just watched as my would-be "rescuee" held his ground and eventually sent his tormenters into silence.

On the bus ride the next day, I sat next to these two mysterious newcomers. "You know, yesterday, I was just trying to help," I told the exclamation point. "I know," he said, "but you didn't need to. We had it handled." He then introduced himself by his nickname, Digger, and revealed that his seatmate was his older brother, James. A fan of the TV show *Dallas*, he told me, his grandmother had called him after her favorite character, Willard "Digger" Barnes, at an early age, and the name had stuck ever since. I found this amusing, given I had been told that my mother loved the name Blake, thanks to Blake Alexander Carrington from the TV show *Dynasty*. By the end of the bus ride, we were all friends, learning that we had more in common than any of us had probably ever imagined.

By the start of junior high school, I became a regular guest at the Wells' house, much preferring their home environment to my own. Their father, Mickey, was a tough, short-tempered man who worked several odd jobs around town, but beneath the fiery exterior, he was a kind and loving man. The gentle and guiding heart of the family came from their mother, Lisa, a joy-filled and quiet woman who seemed to have a smile permanently etched across her face. They would do everything together, which meant there was always something to do or happening in their home, and they were never bothered that I made myself something of an unofficial family member over time. It was through my time at the Wells household that I began to redefine my understanding of *family*, one of the core pillars of my life today. Family didn't have to be flesh and blood; it could be any group of people that you respected, trusted, and loved, and vice versa.

While I still had my responsibilities at home, as long as Mom was off or Poppa could watch Crystal, then Mickey and Lisa didn't seem to mind picking me up and driving us all to the skating rink or taking me along on their family vacations. Additionally, anytime their church had youth activities, they would ensure that if I could go, I was with them at the event. I also got to see my dad every Friday, and we would be allowed to stay the night every other Friday. These grew into nights on which Digger and James became frequent guests as well. My dad and Mickey slowly became friends over the course of the next several school years, having seen so much of each other during pick-ups and drop-offs at one place or the other. It also wasn't long before I learned that both Digger and James were accomplished wrestlers, which was probably why they weren't too concerned about a group of mouthy bullies on the bus that day. I was curious about their wrestling activities, but my schedule with Crystal had never allowed me to truly participate in sports. Then, in my eighth-grade year, Poppa worked it out to be able to stay a few hours later than normal, allowing me to attend practice as long as I came straight home once it was over. Lisa told Mickey that I might like to go to James and Digger's wrestling practice. "Well, we will get the boy or take him home if he wants to go," Mickey told her.

The next thing I knew, I was in the cellar below our school's gymnasium. I still remember the thickness of the humidity and the rubber mats, the sounds of slapping, heavy thuds, and screams of both pain and excitement echoing throughout the cinderblock building. Coach Chang patrolled the outer bounds of the room with a whistle. While Digger and James began warming up, Mickey walked to Coach Chang and began speaking to him. After a few seconds, he waved for me to come over to them.

"Coach says it's OK with him if you want to practice with these boys today, get a feel for it. What'd you say?"

I had only ever been on a couple of rec league sports teams in my life, so I spent a few seconds in silent bewilderment.

"*Well?*" Mickey urged.

"Yeah … um … yes, sir! But what do I do?"

I changed into some shorts and, not having a pair of wrestling shoes, walked onto the mat in my socks. I began to warm up alongside Digger and James, relying on them to help me learn the ropes. I don't know what it was exactly—the first feeling of belonging to something, perhaps, or maybe some inexplicable natural ability for the sport—but I was surprisingly good. I knew how to follow commands and didn't mind doing so. I knew how to be an adult, so to speak, or at least how to please them well enough to keep them off my back. But more than anything, I didn't want to jeopardize this opportunity to belong to something. I would have done anything to prolong that feeling, so I did.

By my freshman year of high school, I was among the best wrestlers in my region and began taking the sport seriously. I trained every day year-round and found a new identity. "I'm a wrestler," I told myself. I wore my letterman jacket all the time, with all my medals for various tournament wins decorating the entirety of the front of the jacket. Throughout high school, James devoted his time to developing automotive skills through shop classes and customizing his truck, while Digger and I continued to wrestle and slowly became known as two of the best wrestlers not only in our school but in our regional conference as well, often winning or at least getting on the podium at all the major tournaments. Additionally, this created a way for me to see my father more, as he became my biggest fan and attended every match.

While high school isn't a particularly enjoyable experience for most teenagers, it was surprisingly the happiest stretch of time I'd ever had in my life up to that point.

As graduation approached, James moved into the workforce while Digger and I decided we would try to attend the same college. This was not an easy task. Coming from low-income families, we both needed to find the best solution. We visited Longwood College together, a small college later turned university, a few hours northeast of Martinsville. While there, we learned of various federal programs that provided either grants or loans. Unfortunately, my mother made about $32,000 per year, which of course was about $2,001 above the cutoff for the grants, so getting a loan in my name was the only option. The next fall, Digger and I headed off to a college dormitory together, leaving James and Crystal and our small town behind.

It wasn't long before Digger and I decided that a schedule that included two wrestling practices per day and traveling to other schools for meets several weekends each semester was cramping our idea of the college experience.

As the end of our first semester approached, we both decided to quit the team. However, our coach stepped in and offered me a scholarship if I agreed not to quit. I agreed and went to work trying to reduce the amount of loans I knew I was going to have to repay. Digs and I had been inseparable since that day on the bus in fourth grade, but our priorities were beginning to differ. The party lifestyle led him down a path to drink more, skip classes, and stay out late more frequently. Don't misunderstand me; I was also caught up in the whirlwind of drinking and partying, but I was begrudgingly forced to limit my fun every week due to practices and tournaments. This made it far more challenging for me to balance the responsibilities of being a member of the wrestling team. I knew I was having less fun and was more tired than Digger. Nonetheless, I pushed forward, trying to balance both.

Nearly halfway through that spring semester, both my team's and my efforts paid off, as we became Division II and III tristate champions. This has always been impressive to me for two reasons. First, we did not have a complete roster, yet we had someone in over half of the individual weight class finals; if you considered the consolation brackets, we dominated as a school. In fact, most of us were individual champions of our own classes as well. Second was just how hard the team pushed one another. It was truly an atmosphere of iron sharpens iron. The last half of the semester, I was able to refocus my effort on enjoying the, shall we say, less-disciplined aspects of the college experience.

Before our sophomore year, Digger was placed on academic probation for one semester, and the possibility that he would not return to school became clear and proved true by the beginning of the coming fall semester. As strange as it may sound, I was only saddened that Digger and I would not continue this journey together. I was well acclimated to isolation, so I felt relatively unmoved by the aloneness of the circumstances. Self-sufficiency was the single emotion I most understood. It felt like home.

I continued to wrestle, but realizing the nearly nonexistent options to wrestle for a livelihood, I began to lose interest in both wrestling and my studies. As they had with Digger, Longwood administrators eventually decided to place me on academic probation at the end of my junior year. I returned to Martinsville that summer and took a job that my stepmother, Teri, helped me get at Fieldcrest, a textile mill. I also began hanging out with James and Digger again, as they had both stayed in town.

I lived for about a year in a rundown apartment with Derrick Ingram, who had been a loosely associated friend but quickly grew to be a new brother in my extended family while we both worked in the loading docks at Fieldcrest. In short order, I performed well enough in my role that I became a shift supervisor within months. My youthful ego soon got the best of me, however, as I quit this supervisory position in order to respond to, what I thought was, a high-paying job in sales. I was going to try my hand at selling vacuum cleaners door-to-door, of all things, which did not pan out as I had imagined. About three months into this venture, my father intervened in disgust. "If you're going to quit school and live here, you can't live like this," he told me.

He arranged a job interview for me at the Pulaski Furniture warehouse, where he was the senior manager. I admit that when I first started working there, I slacked. I took long breaks, moved slowly, and was, in every sense of the word, a bum. In time, that would change. One day, it just clicked in me; I understood who I was to everyone I worked with. I thought about my dad and his faith in me. From that point on, I didn't want to be the boss's son who came in late and hungover, sleeping through my breaks and not taking my opportunities seriously. I wanted to be someone he was proud of, not embarrassed by. I buckled down from that moment on. I came in early, left late, and did every job that needed to be done without needing to be asked or told. The reality was, I was embarking on a career that I'd never intended to pursue but would ultimately excel in, even against my most fantastical visions.

One weekend night, I attended a party at a former high school classmate's house. The host introduced me to a girl named Julie, who happened to be home from a nearby all-women's college for Christmas break. Julie had allegedly told our mutual friend that she thought I was attractive. Unbeknownst to me, our friend had told Julie that I'd said the same about her. It's not that either of us thought her comments weren't true, but our mutual friend was playing both sides without our knowledge. A modern-day cupid, you might say.

By the time Julie went back to college a month later, we were in a serious relationship. We talked every day, and I would drive to Sweet Briar College to see her as often as I could. Three months after we began dating, Julie and I were at a crossroads. She was pregnant. I was twenty-three, Julie was only twenty, and while we had only known each other for a short time, we knew we had something special together. Not knowing who else to turn to, I went to my dad for advice. He told me I should marry her. Julie and I agreed, and that afternoon, my stepmother took Julie to buy a dress at a boutique in town. A pastor friend of my father's only agreed to officiate our wedding as a favor to my father—I only recently learned that he waited to mail the certificate until the last possible moment—and just like that, we were married before dinner. Now, I know what you may be thinking. But after nearly twenty-four years of marriage (at the time of this book's publishing), we are still together, best friends, and our love for one another is stronger than ever.

Around the same time that we found out Julie was pregnant, I was fortuitously promoted to a supervisor position in an eight-hundred-thousand-square-foot warehouse. I was immediately given the "Bad News Bears" team, presumably as a test to see if I could handle it. After developing a warehouse organizational system in which we spray-painted storage sections with specific colors, letters, and numbers to help workers find products faster and more easily, we were the most productive and least error-ridden team in the warehouse. Did I do that? No, I was too young to lead, so I simply created an environment that we all wanted to be in. There was no one person better than the other, and when work needed to be completed, they knew I would be shoulder to shoulder trying to outwork them, which they wouldn't allow.

With my new impromptu career came doubts about why, or even if, I should return to Longwood. I was making more money than I ever had before, and I had a stable job with an open promotion track in front of me. The idea of going back to school just didn't seem logical. I knew that going away to sit through classes I had no interest in would absolutely not be a good idea for me. I knew I would cruise along and fall back into my party lifestyle. This career felt more like wrestling; I had stumbled onto something I was surprisingly good at, something that gave me a rare sense of pride and belonging. So, I decided to stay in Martinsville to continue my job training and attempt to move my way up in the field of supply chain logistics.

Eight months after our wedding, our daughter, Lucy, was born. I felt as though I had stumbled into a career, a marriage, and fatherhood in the blink of an eye, and, in many ways, I had. But emotionally, I still felt strangely numb. I wasn't unhappy; I just didn't feel the type of euphoric emotions I'd heard others describe. I only thought about the duties and responsibilities I had stretched out before me; once again, I began to imagine how things should be and simply tried to make them reality.

Having my daughter didn't give me the confidence I was lacking at the time. That would have required me to know what I must do, and I had no clue. But knowing that I was a father gave me an incredible sense of resolve not to be what many people in my town had often called some of my friends growing up: trailer park trash, or TPT for short. I now had the opportunity to create the family I had always wished to be a part of, and nothing was going to mess that up, certainly not me. She would not be branded TPT, not my little girl.

I quit drinking, partying, and hanging out with anyone and everyone who might interfere with my ability to be what I thought was the best husband and father I could be, including my extended family of Digger, James, Derrick, and Benjamin (a high school classmate with whom I rekindled a connection during my sophomore year at Longwood). I threw myself into my job. I remember how proud I felt to be going to work in khakis and a dress shirt, as opposed to my worn-out jeans and old T-shirts. By the end of that year, I was promoted to a different branch of the company called Ridgeway Clocks, which had a different location nearby but was still a division of Pulaski Furniture.

Once again, I was faced with a new challenge as the continuous improvement manager. My job was to walk the facility and observe the manufacturing process and come up with new ways to find cost savings. I began walking the grounds and seeking out the folks who had been doing the job for quite some time. I observed them, but, more importantly, I asked them questions with humility and sincerity about what would make their jobs easier. Then I listened to them. In less than a year's time, simply by listening to my team's feedback, we were able to collectively produce more than $1 million of annualized savings together.

In January 2003, after roughly one year of me being in this position, my father saw an ad in the paper that he felt I should respond to. At the time, Pulaski's VP of operations, Gene, had left the company to work for a global supply chain company. Gene had been a terrific example to me and took me under his wing early on to help mentor me. "This looks like the place Gene may have gone to work. You should call them," Dad said. I started working on my résumé and applied.

My initial interview was held on-site at the client's location in Virginia. I was interviewed first by the owner of the company and then by the customer for whom I would be providing services. During the interview, I asked, "Is there a Gene that works here?" With a slightly perplexed look, the owner, Andre, sat up and said, "No, he does not, but why do you ask?" I proceeded to explain my role and how we had worked together for my former employer. Shortly after the interview, I learned that the two did know one another and that Gene's response was simply, "Hire that kid immediately."

I remember getting a call offering me the job before that week had ended. But there was one catch: I would have to travel to the corporate office for one week of training. This was new to me and not the kind of expense that funds were readily available to cover. So, after some discussion, Julie and I called my potential future boss, Andre, to ask if I would be compensated for the gas and lodging. "Are you kidding me?" he asked, enraged. "I just gave you a job and you're worried about the travel expense? Are you serious right now?"

Twenty-three, naïve, and desperate, I nearly choked on my own tongue. I wanted to slap myself for even asking a question that, in retrospect, wasn't *that* outrageous but, at the time, felt like the dumbest thing I'd ever said. Of course I was worried about the cost of my travels. I only had a few hundred dollars in the bank, with a wife and baby at home. We did not have funds for a weeklong vacation, much less for me to cover the costs of going and staying three states away for a week with no pay, but I knew it had to be done.

"No. I'm sorry. It's not a problem," I said reluctantly. "I have it covered." It was another lesson in following instructions not because I believed they were right but because I knew that by doing so, I would avoid unwanted and ambiguous punishment. In most cases, you know more than you know. In this instance, I did for sure, so I rolled the dice, took the job, and paid for the travel arrangements myself.

I spent a week in the corporate office soaking up everything I could, watching every move my peers made. I never spoke unless spoken to and always made sure that I understood enough about a task to be able to figure it out on my own as much as possible. I wanted to prove that I was a hard worker and would be little trouble and inconvenience for anyone else. At the end of the week, Andre walked up to my desk and tossed an envelope onto it. "That should cover your expenses," he said before walking away. Having not provided any type of expense report, I was anxious to see how much was on the check. When he was out of view, I quickly opened it to peek and found that he had given me something like fifteen hundred dollars. What the exact amount was, I'm not sure, but I do remember thinking it more than covered my gas and a week's stay at a nearby Hampton Inn. It was the largest single check that I'd ever seen up to that point.

I called Julie as soon as I got on the road going home, telling her that I had a good feeling about the new job while doing my best to contain the adrenaline pumping through me. I drove through the night back to Martinsville, fueled by the elation I felt for our future's potential—a foreign feeling to me at the time. Julie and I celebrated, dancing with young Lucy in our little apartment, only half knowing that our lives would never be the same.

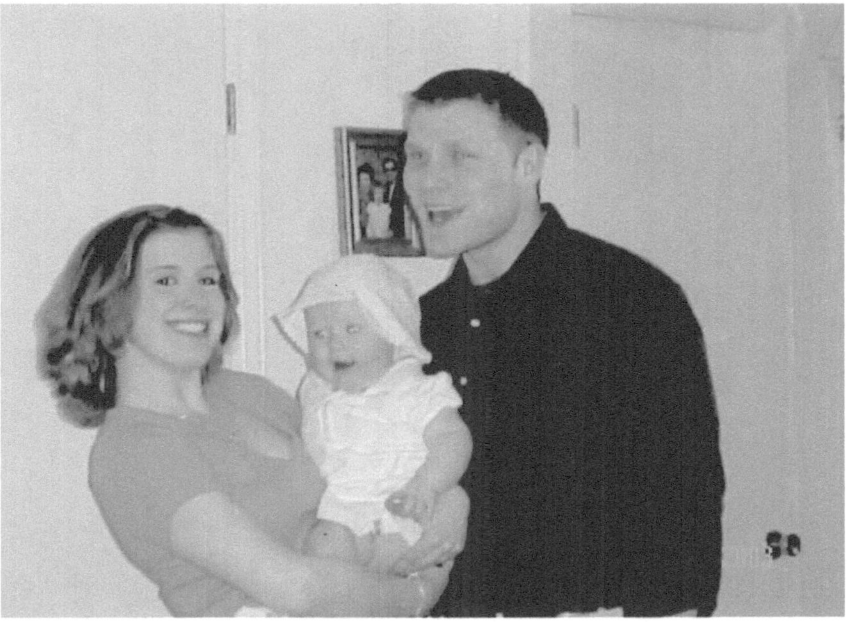

CHAPTER TWO
UNCERTAINTY

SUMMER 2016

I can still remember the sounds of our feet on the trail, the wind blowing through the bright green canopy of the poplars, pines, and sycamores above us. I remember the sun on my face and the sweat and exhilaration of pushing beyond my limits only to find more on the other side.

Our local office had a team of roughly fifty people now, and four of us had spent the year dedicating an hour and a half daily to our own workout routine. We alternated between twelve-mile runs through the wooded trails near our office and doing ninety minutes of the P90X exercise program. On our running days, I remember returning to the office, sweating and full of adrenaline, to then pick off the ticks that covered each other's backs and legs.

Andre had just completed the sale of the NEWCO to a private equity firm a few months before the summer of 2016 rolled into Martinsville. The sales figure was astonishing, our culture and work–life balance was excellent at the time, and everyone came to the office in a great mood, ready to work. We felt like a family, and I was on cloud nine about what we managed to accomplish.

As summer came to an end, I decided to take a break from working out so vigorously and didn't run again until November. Having gone from running seventy-plus miles a month to logging no miles at all so abruptly, I started back slowly, only running two or three miles at a time. The first few times I ran, I had this strange feeling in my legs unlike anything I'd ever experienced. It felt like a sonar pulse moving up my legs in short waves, no more than two or three seconds at a time.

Throughout the month of November, I chalked it up to another byproduct of getting older and having not run in two months, and I tried to stretch more and run more often. The more I ran, though, the more frequently the sensation occurred, although just as fleetingly each time. From December through January, I switched to running on a treadmill indoors, and yet the sensation still came occasionally. It didn't occur every time I ran, maybe a few times over those three months, but the feeling was so foreign to me that each time it happened, it stuck in my mind for days.

I had been seeing a chiropractor for a few years because of two compressed vertebrae, so I thought I might have pinched a nerve and just needed an adjustment. I went to my friend and chiropractor for the adjustment and proceeded to explain the sensations. Several minutes into adjusting my spine, he stopped and stared at me, his face deep in thought. "What?" I asked him. "You know, Blake, this doesn't sound like it would be related to your vertebrae issues. It does make me think you should monitor this closely. The fact is, I don't know what's going on exactly, but let's try a few more simple tests and go from there." He proceeded to conduct a series of tests on me by tapping on the bottoms of my feet and knees to assess my reflexes, concluding that nothing was wrong with my body's response systems and that there was no clear indication of what may be causing the behavior. *I'm in control,* I thought. *I'm in the best shape of my life—physically, mentally, emotionally. I have little to no stress. Nothing is wrong. All I need to do is work harder.*

I left his office vowing to continue getting adjustments and to increase my exercise regimen, convinced that the pulsing would go away eventually and that nothing was wrong. All I needed to do, I thought, was continue to outrun, outwork, and outthink it by creating a new image of health in my head and then making that a reality. I was in complete control of my life and body, and nothing could override that, not now.

CONTROLLING THE CIRCUMSTANCES

When Crystal was a child, a balloon popped in her face. It startled her so badly that she remained afraid at the very sight of a balloon for years. I saw an opportunity in this fear and began tying balloons to doorknobs, walls, or cabinet doors to keep her from doing things she wasn't supposed to do or going places she wasn't supposed to go. It was one of the first lessons I taught myself—how to use an environment or circumstance to produce a desired result. The first time I returned home from college, she was wearing a balloon around her wrist, smiling ear to ear, as if to say, "Look, I'm not afraid anymore."

My life has come with a lot of uncertainty, from childhood to my present life living with MS. Perhaps it's been that lifetime of uncertainty about what the future will hold that produced my ability to remain calm and focused, determined to control everything I could about my environment. I needed to know that I could control as much as possible to relieve my anxiety about what the future might drag into my life. I could direct the environment around Crystal like a symphony conductor, and I learned to please my mother's every peccadillo so I could enjoy a few hours of peaceful freedom each night. But controlling my environment as a young, working father and husband did not come as easily. I struggled to evenly divide my time and attention between work and family. At the time, I believed that being a good husband and father meant succeeding in my career. After all, staying out of the trailer parks and crummy, cramped apartments seemed like the best thing I could do for my wife and daughter. That required me to put nearly all my waking hours and energy into climbing the ranks at work.

Back in 2003, at FIRSTCO (effectively, the first iteration of the NEWCO), I had been assigned to an account local to my area. My initial role was a kind of on-site consultant, charged with providing general shipping and logistics support to them in-house. I'm curious by nature and like to feel useful. I began using my furniture and process improvement experience to work with the employees to improve their job functions. Within months, I was working with my customer's upper management team to find ways to cut costs (even to my own employer), harness new technologies to create more efficiency in production and distribution, and a variety of other things. It was during this time that I taught myself the basics of coding and building customizable workflows using Visual Basic and Microsoft Excel. Through this new skill set, I redesigned the internal tools my customer used to order new products. This one task was optimized from a five-day process down to a forty-five-minute wait time and, ultimately, down to the press of a button.

Less than a year after joining FIRSTCO, I told myself that the only way I could move past a senior supervisor role might rely on whether I had some sort of college degree. So, I enrolled in night and online classes after asking an advisor, "What piece of paper can I get quickly if I transfer my Longwood credits?" Eighteen months later, I completed my bachelor's degree in communications.

With a piece of paper within my grasp and working knowledge of a wide range of functions within the supply chain sector now at my disposal, I asked Andre if I could open and run an office in Martinsville. I was not sure if he thought I was serious, but he replied strongly regardless. "Of course! All you need to do is handle enough business to justify the cost." Because FIRSTCO was a relatively small and young company and I had been one of its early hires, I had the good fortune of enjoying a long leash and was allowed to take on responsibilities above my pay grade, so to speak, if I wished.

The first thing I did was build an environment that would control my behavior, remember the sequence of events, and mitigate exposure to costly mistakes. I named this creation the "Database." Next, I needed accounts. I was a long distance away from the main office, so I got to know everyone by helping them with their more complex accounts. I would call them nearly every day, saying, "Hey, I finished that job already, and I'm bored. You got anything else I can do? Just show me how to do it, and I'll take care of it." It didn't take long before the simple thing to do was to let me run the account.

After diving into operations and picking up my first couple of accounts, I learned of a guy in the corporate office, Neo, who was the first person Andre had hired when he founded FIRSTCO and was, perhaps, in my opinion, the single best operator in our industry. While the average person in his position processed eight hundred to one thousand containers per year, Neo was handling more than ten thousand containers every year by himself. I wanted to know how he was able to balance the chaos of that many shipments, so I got his number and called him directly.

"Hey, Neo, I'm starting to work on and manage accounts now and was wondering if I could come down and shadow you."

"No one has ever asked me that before," he said, laughing.

"Is that a yes, then?"

"Sure, come on down."

When I arrived at the corporate office, I learned that Neo got to his office at five thirty every morning, shut his door, and didn't allow anyone to enter until eleven that morning. He would cuss you out and/or make you eat a foreign cookie if you violated this rule; but, thankfully, he allowed me to bring in a stool and sit, quiet as a bird, in the corner of the room to watch what he did and take notes. He was so unforgiving about this rule that after a week of everyone seeing me in his office without being kicked out, I could sense a difference in how everyone in the office was looking at and treating me. It was as though I could sense the respect the others had for me now, or at the very least, that they were impressed that Neo would allow me in his office so early and repeatedly without him considering it a violation of his own rules.

It was during this time that I observed how Neo's process was not only different from everyone else's but also how he did everything manually. He wrote everything in pen and used physical folders for each shipment. Although his knowledge and skill set towered above others, it looked like a nightmare and a recipe for disaster should anything happen to that office.

When I returned to Martinsville, I immediately began thinking about how to translate the manual steps into something that could be monitored easily and include controls to lower errors within my

Database. After many long nights and weekends, I was able to design the functionality that would optimize effort and time. Once completed, I immediately began consolidating the work for any account I was either managing or processing for my coworkers.

I knew the foundations were being laid to open my own office. I also believed I needed more accounts to accomplish this. I went out to my local region and began to find new clients, beginning with my old employer, Pulaski Furniture. In time, I was beginning to close in on managing ten thousand containers per year on my own. Since I was not in the home office, security dictated that I not have my own username and access to our system. This meant no freight moved under my name. This also meant I would need to input someone else's name for any new accounts. To continue on this path of building a new reality, I didn't want to slow down, so I created all new accounts under Neo's name.

After some time, Andre asked Neo what was going on, congratulating him for the new accounts and his ability to balance so many of them. "It's not me. It's Blake. Go talk to him," Neo told him. It should be noted that I was working sixty to eighty hours a week on a salary of $26,000 per year, leaving little time in my life for anything else. Meanwhile, Julie and Lucy were bonding at home as Lucy entered her toddler years. We were still scraping by, even though Julie was also contributing to our family by working at a local credit union. I wasn't certain that all my accomplishments at work were going to receive any recognition, as they were technically being logged under Neo's name. But one day, out of the blue, Andre called me and told me that he had heard what I was doing and was going to give me a raise, effective immediately. That further incentivized me for two reasons: I knew that I could trust Andre and Neo to acknowledge my efforts and that I would be rewarded for them.

Within two years, I had opened a branch in Martinsville, and using six of the companies eighty-plus employees, we became the most efficient location and managed over 60 percent of FIRSTCO's total business. By the time I was twenty-eight, I was making well into six figures, Julie no longer had to work, and we did everything two twentysomethings who had never had anything would do with that kind of money: luxury cars, a new house, expensive clothes, fancy restaurants, etc. At the same time, Julie had become the youth pastor at our church, and our time spent together was increasingly slim.

Andre sold the company to a private equity firm on two separate occasions. The first was simply a partnership for expedited growth. During this time, he moved more into the traditional ownership role, focusing on sales, while our CFO, Gary, took the reins as CEO. Gary eventually flew to Virginia to offer me a promotion to be his COO, which would have required me to work in the corporate office full-time. I turned it down. Now, some of you may be thinking I'm crazy for doing that. Well, another thing that Neo taught me was leverage—its value and who has it. Julie and I had no interest in leaving our new home. I believed that I had the leverage to keep control without moving. However, I also believed if I turned down the position, then they might go outside of the company to hire, and that would not be good for anyone.

At the time, I was working closely with a new hire, Lionel, taking on Andre's operational responsibilities, especially while Andre was handing off his final daily touchpoints. This evolved into conversations in which Andre focused on sales, Lionel on routings, and I on execution. We three made a great team, and I didn't want this to change, either. I knew if I recommended Lionel, then he and I would continue to run the day-to-day business together, and I wouldn't have to move. So, I recommended my new friend and colleague. I assured each member of the new executive team of Lionel's ability and, more importantly, how we would communicate with each other to run the organization.

Initially, this was easier for Gary to accept than it was for Gene, who by this point had also joined our company as one of the members of the executive management team. Gene called immediately to voice his disappointment with my response but affirmed that he would continue to support and trust my decision. For a short while, this allowed me to continue my accustomed levels of control without the barrage of bureaucracy weighing me down. As a bonus, Lionel and I developed into a great working team within the world of supply chain and logistics.

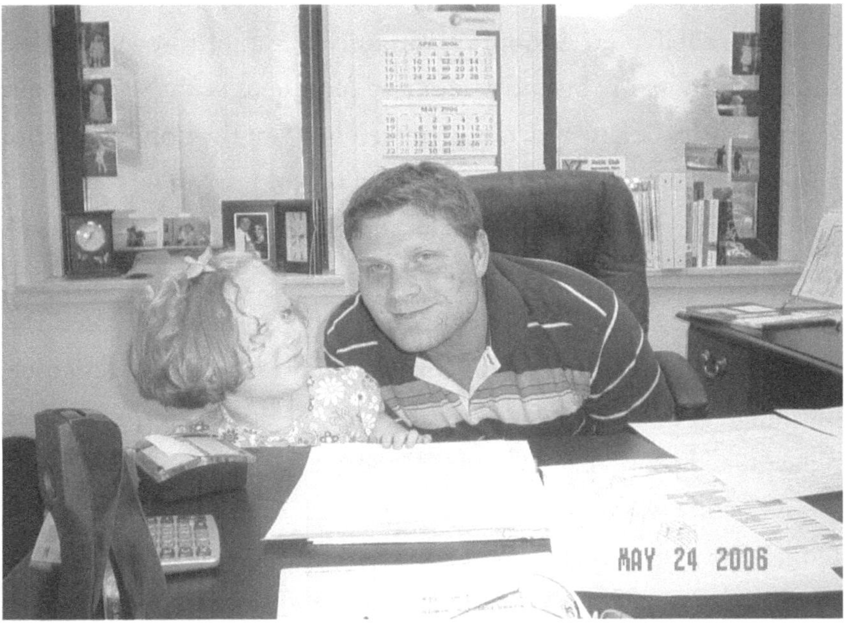

By 2007, the company completed its second sale and was under the full ownership of a private equity group. The old management was out, and a completely new group entered. This group was beginning to ruin the culture of the company we had worked so hard to create. A small segment of us began questioning the decisions being forced on us; the justification for why the changes were happening was not driven from a place of logic. We knew we could do it better. Thus, we started another logistics company, which I'll refer to simply as "the NEWCO."

Once again, I paid for my travel arrangements to take on a new adventure. This time, I knew on whose expense and risk this venture would be. I camped out on Lionel's couch; he was also part of the founding group. Our task was simple: build an environment with minimal expenditures, push to expand margin while maintaining positive cash flow, and develop strong customer retention. We knew if we were able to sustain this for two years, then not only would Andre be eligible (and more importantly, ecstatic) to own another successful company but he would also reunite us with Neo and our winning team. That idea was a tremendous motivation, and quite honestly, two years is not a long time in our industry.

We got to work. Of course, my contribution to our group wasn't my ability to fund the start-up monetarily. I earned my equity through sweat by mitigating the costly operational errors that plagued the larger corporate offices at our previous employer. I began designing, building, and executing the creation of all operating procedures, policies, and processes; thus, the "Database 2.0" was born. Once the infrastructure was in place, I returned home. After finding a location, Lionel drove up and joined me for an eventful eve as we opened the company's first office location in Martinsville. The first day proved to be eventful as well, or at least something I should have seen coming. The first call that came through our new 1-800 number was from none other than Gene, telling me how disappointed he was in my decision to leave. The past and future of my life and career were diverging, but taking his call forced me to see the beginning of that break very clearly.

I was now playing a much larger role. My oversight extended to all global operations, technology, and people. I became obsessed with process and rules. I often spoke harshly to the team, expected everyone to work long hours until the job was done, and I never "logged off" from work at home. When I got there, I would often sit silently, even at the dinner table, and then go to my office to work on my computer until one or two o'clock in the morning. In time, working without sleep became a frequent fixture of my schedule as well.

I didn't intend to be rude or coarse with anyone, but I treated everyone like they were Crystal in some ways. I thought I had to explain everything slowly and control every environment I was in—every person and every task—to ensure that the results would satisfy me. One day, I got a call from my friend Lionel, and he said it to me straight. "Hey, everyone says you're being an asshole. You have to stop being an asshole."

I sometimes see parts of myself in the character Sheldon Cooper from *The Big Bang Theory*, in that I'm not great at navigating social interactions gracefully. I'm direct and logical, and by nature, I struggle to understand how to speak to others in any other way, so I had to train myself to remain calm and try to understand why someone might be struggling with something before speaking to them. I had to get outside of my own head more and consider the strengths, weaknesses, and preferences of personalities different from mine in order to be a better boss and leader. It was an incredible challenge for me but ultimately one that I overcame.

Unfortunately, I only overcame those flaws in the workplace and was unable to translate it to my homelife with Lucy and Julie, where I remained very practical, matter-of-fact, and at times impatient and controlling. If I was idle, I would think ahead to what I needed to do next or to what more I could have done that day. I had programmed myself to have no off switch. I even trained my teams to be sure they did everything they could think of every single day and to not leave until we couldn't think of anything else that needed to be done. I was burying myself in work because I was so good at it, and because I was good at it, I kept getting rewarded for it. It became a cycle that ultimately led to an imbalance of priorities in my life. I was never really present because I kept my mind trained on the future. God, however, would soon have different plans for me that I would ultimately have no control over at all.

CHAPTER THREE
A TICKING TIME BOMB

SPRING 2017

The first time I lost feeling in my body was a calm Saturday afternoon. I was relaxing on the bed when I realized that I couldn't feel parts of my torso. I rolled over only to discover that my entire left side was, in fact, numb. After a few minutes, I began to feel that deep tingling sensation, like you get after sitting on your foot too long just before the feeling returns to normal. After the tingling faded, the feeling in my side returned to normal.

On Sunday morning, I woke up and went to use the bathroom, as I usually do first thing. I was shocked when I realized everything was completely numb "down there," and feeling didn't return to the region until close to an hour later. I simply chalked it up to aging and thought little else about it. If nothing else, I could see that I needed the rest that weekend.

On my drive to work Monday morning, however, I felt this tingling on the left side of my face before the sensation traveled like a shock wave down my left arm. The feeling was strong enough that I veered my car off to the side of the road and stopped, believing that I was having some sort of a stroke or heart attack. *Am I going to die right here?* I thought. I turned around and drove myself to the emergency room (ER). I rushed to the front desk and told them I thought I might be having a stroke or a heart attack and wanted to be tested immediately. I was escorted to the back, where I explained my symptoms to multiple doctors who each showed signs of perplexed concern.

"We need you to come with us," one of them told me. I was immediately whisked away into a large, humming cylinder where I heard voices giving me directions through an intercom to remain as still as possible. After a few minutes, they pulled me out of the machine and told me to wait in a little nook in the ER while they processed my results. It seemed like years passed by in a blurry mixture of anxiety, denial, panic, and optimism. "Maybe it's just something to do with my compressed vertebra, a little nerve thing," I told myself. After a couple of hours, the sound of the curtain shrieking open shook me from my emotional roller coaster. A doctor stood in front of me, staring at a clipboard of papers. "OK, Mr. Shumate. Your results so far look promising. We will send everything to your primary care physician (PCP). They will follow up with you further, but it doesn't look to be anything serious, and there's no need to keep you here."

I remembered that I was supposed to fly to Houston the next day, so I asked him if it was safe for me to fly. "Oh, absolutely," he replied. The next day, a Tuesday, I flew to Houston to meet with clients and returned on Thursday. First thing Friday morning, I received a call from my PCP. "Blake, we need you to come in immediately." My concern returned instantly. I practically floated to his office, my mind churning with the possibilities of what the request was about.

He brought me straight into a room and offered me a seat, my file already open in his hand. "I'll cut right to the chase, Blake. These results look like you've either had some sort of stroke or that you're about to have a brain aneurysm. I wanted to talk to you quickly before you did anything crazy, like jump on a plane, since I know you travel a lot. If you fly, this could rupture and kill you." I burst out laughing. "I just got back from Houston last night. That's four flights. I asked this question on Monday for this reason." He shook his head slightly and looked at me seriously. "I'm not saying that's what it is. I'm telling you what these results make me think. These scans don't look good, and I don't want you flying anywhere, as a precaution."

I headed home, unsure of what to believe. The ER's tests were dismissive of anything serious, while my own doctor didn't know if I'd had a stroke or an aneurysm. The uncertainty, the dread of not knowing what's actually happening to you, is an awful feeling, but I wasn't panicked. My mind seemed to instinctually shrug off the symptoms, rationalizing that the inconclusive results and contradiction of it all meant that it was most likely nothing and would pass in time.

When I walked through the door, I called for Julie and began telling her the news. The more I told her, the more concerned she became. Julie did her best to stay calm, but she was stunned and scared. "Is it cancer? Could you have a brain aneurysm while you're driving and die? Could you induce a brain aneurysm by thinking too hard about it? But shouldn't you be thinking about it, considering the options? Have you made a will? Should we?" I held her immediately. I knew she needed to understand my perspective. "I overreacted, and clearly there is nothing wrong nor anything to panic about. No one thinks anything is serious. Otherwise I would be hospitalized. Not to mention I've flown multiple times, which should have killed me if something was really wrong," I said. She listened, and I tried to comfort her fears with my logic. We talked through her concerns until she was calm.

As expected, all of this was forgotten over the following weeks. All my regular routines were in full swing, and life was blissful once again. On a random Friday evening, Julie and I were sitting upstairs watching a movie, distracting ourselves from the day's events. Julie asked me a question about the movie, and when I answered, her eyes widened. I didn't hear it or feel any different than I had all day, but I was slurring my words as though I were heavily intoxicated. Julie, alarmed now, sat up and stared at me. "What are you doing?" she exclaimed. "What are you talking about?" I said, sitting up now too. "Your speech … it sounds like you're drunk. You're slurring your words so much I can hardly understand you."

Now, we were both fully terrified. Julie jumped up and told Lucy to get dressed, and together we put on our shoes, grabbed the keys, and headed to the car. I believed at this point that I was really dying, so we decided that it wasn't worth going five minutes down the road to a small ER that had already given us a reason to doubt their expertise. Instead, we rolled the dice and made the thirty-five-minute drive to a larger hospital.

We arrived around eleven thirty in the evening and ran to the front desk, frantically explaining what was happening. While Julie and Lucy sat in the waiting room, they rushed me back to their ER and ran some preliminary tests. From my perspective, I could see that their silence meant the tests were showing some issues, like they either weren't sure or did know but weren't telling me what those issues were. Instead, they quickly checked me in and got me online with a neurologist. For the next few hours, I talked to this neurologist through a telemedicine program about my symptoms and the tests I'd had so far. They asked me a long list of questions as well, but unfortunately, they could not make any conclusions other than that I needed to have more tests conducted immediately.

A CONCLUSION OF UNKNOWNS

The doctors shipped me off in an ambulance to the nearest dedicated neurology wing, while Julie and Lucy followed in our car. There, I spent two days going through a gauntlet of tests and evaluations conducted by a team of specialists. They began with blood work and performed a spinal tap, various heart tests, more scans, and a litany of other procedures over the course of a single weekend. Still, no one knew exactly what was wrong with me. The only terms being thrown around were the same ones I'd been hearing for a week now: *stroke* and *aneurysm*.

If all these experts and all these tests can't get any closer to an answer than the single scan I had back in Martinsville by an ER physician, how badly off am I? I thought. *Am I the carrier of some undiscovered disease, a real patient zero? Am I a medical anomaly? A freak?* My mind sputtered and raced, flashing images of myself locked in a glass biohazard cube to be studied by scientists in lab coats. Or worse, lying on my deathbed still wondering what was happening to me.

I had avoided doctors as much as I could for most of my life. I have a dangerous personality in that way. If I think I can figure out something relating to my health, I will self-diagnose and create my own plan for how to address it. For better or for worse, I like to do my own research, and I'm convinced that I know my body better than anyone else does. Through my years and years of wrestling, I became very in tune with my body, learning the ins and outs of its limits and how to hear what it was trying to tell me. I had been confident that I would know what it was telling me forever. Considering that I was in the best shape of my life, I had been even more certain of my theory (seriously, I could almost do ten corn cob pull-ups). But now, in addition to the doctors who were supposed to know how to diagnose and treat me, I was doubting myself.

That entire weekend in the hospital, Lucy, Julie, Julie's parents, Joyce and Monroe Young, and my dad and Teri were coming and going, taking turns staying in the room with me to keep me company.

On Sunday evening, a general neurologist came into my room with some long-awaited answers for us. "We have good news for you," he began. "It's not a stroke. You thought it might be a stroke or an aneurysm, but there are lesions on your brain. A lesion is basically a scar left behind after your immune system attacks itself. These lesions harm the sheaths that form around the nerves in your brain called myelin, which act as a kind of insulation around your nerves. Now, I'm not diagnosing you, but all evidence points toward multiple sclerosis, or MS. We're going to set you up for a follow-up consultation and further testing with a neurologist who specializes in this field, but all indications suggest you have multiple sclerosis. Just so you know, MS is an autoimmune-related disease that affects the central nervous system ..."

It felt like the room had begun to spin, and my hearing was dulled by a ringing sound echoing in my ears. The ringing paused when I heard the doctor say, "Unfortunately, MS is hereditary." Upon hearing those words, I broke down. I was sobbing uncontrollably as I thought of Lucy, knowing that she may have some type of autoimmune problem in her lifetime. I also remembered that my mother had been diagnosed with lupus when I was a child. With autoimmune diseases running in my side of the family, Lucy may have to endure the same uncertainty and fear of a disease-altering existence. That thought was more unbearable than the last few weeks of hell I'd been experiencing.

When Digger and I were seniors in high school, we both played on the football team in addition to our time spent on the wrestling mat. Digs had a long history with the coaches and was even one of the captains of our football team, whereas I didn't join until I began driving during my sophomore year. Our coach had taken a liking to us based on our actions both on and off the field. One day, he called us to his office and said that he had a proposition for us.

"I have a disabled friend who could use some help, and he asked me to find two upstanding young men who would be willing to carry him to and from his car every Sunday so he can attend church. It'll only take a few minutes of your time, and he's willing to pay fifty bucks to each of you if you'll do it."

Digger and I just looked at one another, each just as perplexed and excited as the other. "Uh, sure thing, Coach. Absolutely," I said.

"Yeah, no problem, Coach. Be happy to," Digger concurred.

"Great. His name is Dan. Here's his address," Coach Edwards said, scribbling on a sticky note. "Now, he lives on the basement floor of an apartment complex, which is why he needs your help. So you'll have to go to this address and then go into the main entrance. You'll see a set of stairs leading down to his door. Got it?" He handed me the note.

"Yes, sir," we both said. Coach Edwards went on to say something about the disease his friend had, but I was too busy thinking about the fifty bucks, so I really had no idea what he was saying.

When Digger and I arrived at the man's apartment the following Sunday, we were clueless as to what we were going to find on the other side of the door. We knocked and said that Coach Edwards had sent us. Soon, a woman answered the door, introducing herself as Dan's caretaker. "Dan's bedridden," she explained. "He has nurses to put him in his wheelchair during the week, but finding people on the weekend is difficult. Thanks for helping; it makes him so happy to know he has the option to go to church, at least when he feels able to."

She walked us into his bedroom, where we saw a thin, pale man, his hands long and contorted. Just looking at him, I thought he looked too fragile to move. We would have to be very gentle with him. I whispered to Digs that I'd go first, and he could help if I needed him. Digger nodded his head in agreement. I said hello to Dan and told him that I was going to pick him up. I slid my arms under his frail frame and lifted him up. He couldn't have weighed more than a hundred and twenty pounds. I remember how he felt like he was made of jelly. He had little to no muscle mass, and his body draped over my forearms like a thick blanket.

I carried him up the stairs and placed him in the passenger seat of his caretaker's car. Digger and I returned a few hours later, and Digger carried Dan back to his bed. We did this any Sunday that Dan felt like leaving his home, until Digger and I went off to college. All the while, I was certain that Coach Edwards had told me that Dan was suffering from MS.

At the hospital, with the diagnosis of my own MS looming, I thought back to Dan all those years ago. I thought back to that dark basement apartment where his frail and twisted body lay for days on end. I thought about the look in the eyes of a man trapped in a body that would no longer work for him. I thought about the loneliness, the hopelessness, the helplessness of it all. I pondered the pain Dan might have endured when thinking about all the things he would never get to experience for the first time, everything he'd never get to experience again. Then I thought about my future. I thought about all that I might miss. I thought about my own body slipping away until I was a thick blanket draped over a high schooler's arms.

CHAPTER FOUR
TRUTH SEEKER

About six weeks after I was released from the hospital, additional tests by a third neurologist confirmed the suspicions of the first two, and I was officially diagnosed with MS. Further examination found a total of three lesions on my brain. Still, something inside me couldn't accept it. Everything was coming at me so quickly, and the doctors always seemed to be somewhat preoccupied and unwilling to listen to anything I said that didn't match what they wanted to hear. I felt like they were only trying to check me off their list of things to do so they could get to the next blank face on their schedule. I felt like I was on a conveyor belt in an assembly factory at times, moving down a line of workers who—for better and for worse—were only responsible for one specific task before passing the "product" off to the next worker. Whether it was my skeptical nature, dissatisfaction with the care I'd received thus far, or pure shock at what my future might look like, I was determined to get more answers.

I left the hospital preparing for a life living with MS, a disease I still knew almost nothing about. Over the next few weeks, I found myself adjusting to a persistent and gradual loss of control over my body. My ability to engage my legs and arms was deteriorating, as was the degree of sensation in them. My body slowly began to feel like plastic tightly wrapped around a tenderloin. I was struggling to type, and therefore code, or do anything efficiently on my computer, a factor that struck within me great fear and panic surrounding my very sense of worth at work. I began to wrestle with the thought that I may no longer be as independent as I always had been. I may not be able to be "the helper" to people in my life in all the ways I had been; I may now be the one asking for help.

I received my first glimmer of hope when Julie went to check out a new spa for lymph node cleansing and massages in town. She began a conversation with the owner, Ashley, who revealed that she too had been diagnosed with MS several years prior. She described many of the same symptoms I was experiencing. She went on to say that she had been misdiagnosed and actually had Lyme disease, a tick-borne illness with many similar symptoms to MS. Lyme disease is known as the "great mimicker," meaning it presents like many different neurological issues, such as MS and amyotrophic lateral sclerosis (ALS). Therefore, Lyme disease may also cause delayed neurologic symptoms, physical weakness, numbness and pain, fatigue, blurred vision, confusion, and inflammation in the brain and spinal cord. Unlike MS, though, Lyme disease can be treated with antibiotics. If caught early enough, a person with Lyme disease can make a full recovery.

Julie rushed home to relay the news. "Blake!" She was yelling my name even before she came running through the front door. "What, what? Is everything OK?" I said, confused and startled. "I just met a woman who received an MS diagnosis five or six years ago, only it turned out to be a misdiagnosis. It was actually Lyme disease. She began having MS-like symptoms shortly after being bitten by a tick.

That means there's hope. It could be the same for you. Maybe you don't have MS. Maybe it's Lyme disease."

I thought back to the days when I had returned from our runs at work and had to have a coworker pluck from my back five or six ticks at a time. "Wowzers ..." I said, exhaling deeply. I immediately felt a hundred pounds lighter, like I could have floated away. I felt like I had just woken from a nightmare, relieved that it had all just been a dream. There was hope where there hadn't been in more than a month of agony. I had a chance to escape this incurable disease. What had once been the beginning of an unending torment that would forever change my life could just be a mistake. A few weeks or months of antibiotics could reset my body, and I could have my old life back. I could get back to running and working and thinking clearly, to having everything I thought I'd lost restored.

The next day, I made an appointment to see my PCP. When I got in to see him, I didn't even let him say hello. "My wife met a woman recently who was misdiagnosed with MS. She had Lyme disease, which has a lot of early signs that are similar MS. She was bitten by a single tick. I've been bitten by dozens of them. Could this be a simple tick-borne disease rather than MS?" He contemplated for a few seconds and then said, "You may be right. Let me do the test and find out for sure."

This was the end of summer, over a year after my regular twelve-mile runs through tick-infested forests. I had already met with a neurologist who confirmed my MS diagnosis, having rejected the possibility of Lyme disease being the culprit. But no tests had been conducted to definitively prove that I was or was not experiencing Lyme disease or any other tick-borne illness. The hope was that my doctor's test would prove it conclusively one way or the other, but, in hindsight, my desperate pleas for a way out of this newfound horror would never have let me believe a negative test result.

A few weeks later, the results were in, and someone from my PCP's office called to inform me that the test revealed I was negative for Lyme disease. I refused to believe it. Call it optimism, skepticism, or just plain denial, but I didn't trust the results simply because they had been performed by the medical community; there is always room for human or process error. My PCP agreed and repeated the test. But to no avail—the results were the same.

I didn't give up quite yet. I went online and discovered that there is a growing epidemic of tick-borne diseases stretching from the New England region down to the northern portion of South Carolina. Martinsville was in a prime location for such diseases, a hundred miles or so inside the heart of the tick-borne illness heat map. More internet research uncovered a company called IGeneX that specializes in Lyme disease tests. Even better, they accept orders from the public, not just doctors. I mailed in my sample, and a few weeks later, I received the results. Unfortunately, I couldn't interpret them very well, as they were extremely technical. From the markers that I could interpret, there was at least some evidence that I did have Lyme disease, but I could not understand it with complete confidence.

I went back to my PCP and asked if he could refer me to an expert who could help me interpret the IGeneX test results. "Well, there's an infectious disease doctor in Roanoke by the name of Dr. Talty who may be willing to take a look. I don't know her personally, but I'm happy to refer you and see if we can get you in." Shortly after receiving his referral, Dr. Janine Talty's office reached out to set up an appointment for me but informed me that there was a long waiting list and that the first available appointment was not until early the next year, a date roughly six months away. Any answers I was desperately seeking would have to wait, leaving me to chew on the worst possibilities my imagination could conjure for the next half a year.

CHAPTER FIVE
SUPPLY AND DEMAND

FALL–WINTER 1989

By the time I smelled the smoke creeping down the hall, into my bedroom, a quarter of the kitchen was already swirling with orange-and-black flames. I found Crystal just standing there in the middle of the kitchen, coughing uncontrollably and frozen in shock. A game of playing "house" at dawn had gone awry, as the very real dangers of microwaving metal forks had exploded into a nightmarish reality for her and for me. I grabbed her by the shoulders and gently shook her. "Crystal! Crystal, look at me!" Startled, she turned to me wide-eyed and screamed. "Come with me; we have to get outside right now!" I said as I took her by the arm and proceeded to pull her through the kitchen, across the living room, and down the porch onto the front lawn. "Stay here. Do you understand, Crystal? Stay here; don't go back inside!" She looked at me and nodded with her hand on top of her head. I ran back into the house and woke our mother, who was so dead asleep from her twelve-hour shift the night before that she had neither heard the yelling nor smelled the burning plastic, wood, and metal. "Mom, wake up! The house is on fire! The house is on fire! We have to get out!" She squinted an eye open and looked at me in disbelief. "Wha-what are you talking about? What's going on?" I grabbed her by a forearm and began to pull. "The house is on fire. There was an accident in the kitchen, and it's on fire. We have to get out. Come on!" We ran down the hall and outside to Crystal. Mom then took my sister next door to a neighbor's house to call 911. As soon as I dropped Mom off with Crystal, without thinking, I ran back inside and moved the furniture to the other side of the room and grabbed the towels off the freezer. I then immediately ran to the sink and grabbed the fire extinguisher. I went to the entryway to take a deep breath. From there, I just pointed the extinguisher at the flaming wall, and then, with my good eye closed and mouth shut, I squeezed the trigger until I emptied the extinguisher and the flames were beaten back into a small corner, smoldering and no longer stretching across the ceiling. Once I saw no more flames, I retreated outside.

Sirens, lights, and the voices of concerned neighbors began to fill the smoky morning air around us until, an hour or so later, the fire captain declared that the fire had been extinguished and the bulk of the damage was contained only to one wall in the kitchen. "You did good, son. It could've been much worse. You've got a brave boy there," he said to my mother.

It was a month before Thanksgiving, so Crystal and I would be shuffling between my dad's house and my mother's for various family gatherings. Over the next few weeks, my mother's insurance paid to have the carpets replaced, the walls repainted, and new kitchen cabinets and countertops installed (including a childproof microwave). By the time Thanksgiving rolled around, we practically had a new house. Perhaps that played a role in my mother's relatively calm reaction to the fire. Though she was deeply stressed about the damage initially, in time, she began to speak about the entire event as though it amused her.

It was the Saturday before Christmas. My dad came and picked us up so we could spend some of the day with his side of the family at the house of my grandparents, Patsy and Sam Shumate. I was sitting on the floor surrounded by my grandparents, aunts, uncles, and a few of my cousins when my dad came out of a room down the hall with a wrapped, rectangular-shaped object resembling a large picture frame. "Here, Blake," he said through a grimaced grin, stretching his arms out over my cousin's head as the family placed me center stage. "We have one for you." Everyone stopped and watched me, all smiling and eager for me to rip off the paper. I slowly unwrapped it until a framed certificate came into view. The fire department in Roanoke had heard about the fire and arranged for me to be awarded for "heroic action." I was ten years old, and to this day it's one of my most cherished memories. I couldn't have imagined a better gift.

2007–2016

For as long as I can remember, I've always felt like I needed to take care of others. It was, I believed, my duty to do whatever was required of me to protect those who were depending on me. The night of the fire is an example of that mentality, one that I've carried with me as a brother and son, as a husband and a father, as a boss and entrepreneur, as a Christian, and as a friend. I don't know to what degree the fire of '89 played a role in developing that mindset, but I do know it was the first time anyone ever recognized and rewarded me for doing what needed to be done. I'm sure it helped at least a little in setting me on a path to being a protector to those I come across who need one.

When we launched the NEWCO back in 2007, within weeks of returning home after creating the basis of the infrastructure, we opened our first office in Martinsville, Virginia. It was my show to run, and although my equity position was small, I took ownership of every aspect as though it were my business and everyone working there was a member of my family. The processes we developed at my location were implemented at all our other offices. When something wasn't working, I was sent to fix it. Likewise, when something went wrong, everyone got mad at me. But I loved it. I love being challenged. I love being accountable. And I love belonging to a family that I can care for and protect.

My primary role at the company was essentially that of a Swiss army knife, performing various tasks across the organization. I was often called on to fix or develop something operationally, but I also had the task of traveling to visit with existing clients or to meet with potential clients.

For example, Andre, being an economic genius, can spot a rising wave within our industry or beyond to any market-based industry. He would then say, metaphorically, "Here's the wave coming. Make me a surfboard." Such was the case when Andre recognized how far behind the shipping industry was in terms of technology, specifically apps and the offering thereof.

Around 2011, I bought a book from the *How to ... for Dummies* series about how to build apps. I followed the book line by line, built an app, and released it on the App Store two months later. As a result, we became the first non-vessel operating common carrier (NVOCC) to develop a mobile tracking app, and we were riding the media wave, just as Andre had predicted.

By the time 2012 arrived, I had designed and released two additional visibility platforms; however, our big surf would not begin to come in until the summer of that year. Andre was able to find a large beneficial cargo owner (BCO) looking for a supply chain technology partner. The importer was looking for someone to custom build a purchase order management system. After several discussions with their executive team, Andre was certain he could secure the account if we could demonstrate how our technology could deliver this type of service.

As an NVOCC, this opportunity was very rare. This was the single largest account any of us had ever had the opportunity to work with, and what was even more rare was that BCOs of this size typically didn't work with NVOCCs. We were by no means a software company, but Andre believed that, if we were able to give them a website, we may be able to win some of their freight business. When discussing internally, we all knew the opportunity was quoted as an investment, meaning the tech services sold were nonexistent and underpriced. However, the view was that we just needed to get their data online. If we could do that, then we could use the data to pick up some of their ocean freight, which was where we could make the profit to cover the tech start-up costs.

I now had a new purpose, an additional role I could play: lead software developer, so long as I could figure out what that was. I worked through the night for several days, putting together a thirty-five-page document of the systems functionality, visibility, and capabilities of our technology. Essentially, the document was comprised of our company success stories in the form of case studies, awards, and technical highlights of the existing tools I had created for our internal operations, plus a litany of ideas that had not yet come to life. To me, the proposal included every solution and more that they were looking for in a partnership.

Once complete, I drove to meet Andre for an on-site presentation to their management team. I played my part and walked through the proposed solution. Andre continued the negotiations, and he ultimately closed/won the account by committing us to develop and deploy the solution within six months. Now all we had to do was make the proposal real.

For the next several months, it felt like I was back at Ridgeway Clocks. I spent my time on-site, asking questions and learning the differing jobs, roles, departments, and idiosyncrasies of the organization. During this time, our new client assigned a woman named Angela as their company's project manager.

Week in and week out, it felt like Angie and I spent every waking hour working together. During that time, she became a dear friend and one of the most inspirational people I have ever met. She was pregnant with twins while her husband was battling cancer. I was there when her husband ultimately lost his battle, just before she gave birth. Tragically, one of the twins was stillborn. In a matter of weeks, Angie had lost her husband and a child. I couldn't begin to fathom the devastation she was feeling. Miraculously, and to everyone's astonishment, she managed to carry herself with so much grace and strength every single day. For her to navigate that level of heartbreak by focusing on the blessings she still had in her day-to-day life was nothing short of amazing.

Angie and I spent the better part of 2012 building the management system, testing it, and working to process feedback from her organization's staff. One of the biggest problems identified through these discovery sessions was the amount of "he said, she said" bickering among employees and departments. With that in mind, I made it my objective to simply be, well, objective. There was too much emotion in the way teams communicated and shared workloads. So, we designed the system to remove the emotion by capturing the workflow actions and notifying users of their responsibilities and holding them accountable for the lack thereof. Instead of working in silos, users were required to interact with our system for any measurable task, with the goal being to create an auditable systematic process. When or if things were done, everything was recorded. As a result, it didn't matter what someone said they did or didn't do; it only mattered what the system showed them and everyone else.

We deployed the final version of the system in early 2013, and by the end of that year, and thanks to Angie and the great feedback from her team, the system would become one of the best purchase order management tools on the market. As a bonus, because these guys moved over thirty thousand twenty-foot-equivalent units (TEU) annually, we immediately had exposure to hundreds of new importers from around the world; once again, all was happening just as Andre had predicted. He now had all the waves he wanted to ride.

Within months, we blew up as a company. Following the success of building a new purchase order management system, we evolved into designing and building other new contract management programs for other BCOs; each them became best-in-class solutions, all thanks to the honest feedback from the stakeholders involved.

After I had built or designed five or so applications, I thought that I should at least sound like I knew what I was doing. In the fall of 2012, I had enrolled back into school, and, within twenty-four months, I graduated summa cum laude with a degree in software engineering, having clearly seen the need to understand computer technology and coding in our industry.

I didn't have any plans to become a programmer or begin developing apps full-time, but I did want to know if what I was being told by IT professionals made sense or if I should challenge in a greater context with new ideas. Thus far, my experience was proving that many of them liked to speak in jargon, as though they wanted people to think their work was too complex for anyone else to understand. I didn't like that and wanted to be able to call out bologna when I heard it. These apps helped us retain existing business and market our services to expand our reach as a growing company, not to mention streamline many of our operational processes.

In time, I learned that I actually liked to build or fix things, to learn and create. That was my specialty, in fact—my largest value-add to the company. The secret was just doing what I had learned to do in my early twenties while working in furniture warehouses: listen. I just needed to ask the people who would be working with these programs what they were struggling with, what solutions they felt would make their jobs better, and then get to work on finding ways to deliver those solutions to them.

For example, after Andre purchased the company in 2009, a decision was made that we needed to maintain the low overhead costs as we scaled the company. The decision meant that the economics of Martinsville's low wage and rent factors would propel us to be our largest office location. Those same factors also meant that Martinsville was not what you would call a deepwater talent pool. However, by this point, my database creation truncated the supply chain management process into something more of a controlled audit. This allowed us to imagine different ways to create a culture that would provide the desired performance results by leveraging more of a team environment within a solo-performing operations group.

By this point, I already had trusted members of my team who played critical roles in creating such an environment. I built that team by hiring individuals who fit a culture with high levels of integrity and a willingness to work together. Where possible, I would look at open positions as more like seats on a bus, asking questions such as, *What do these people need in a teammate to support our growing culture?*

People such as Rick and Vicky were trusted role players who were highly skilled, proficient in heavy volume, and had great personalities for training others for attitude and success. I also pushed to find opportunities for my extended family members—James, Derrick, and Benjamin—to use their skills to support operations, but I ensured that there were no favorites and that only the best people were in those roles as measured by performance. Ultimately, I had to let many friends go, both new and old, as much as I hated to do it. In time, my team grew and so did my circle of trust as Brad, Lori, John-Michael, Riggs, the cloud team led by Jerry Fackler (a.k.a. J. L. or Worm), and the development team, led by Darren (bringing tech support in-house), all rose to lead their respective divisions. We led the rest of the organization together through a unified approach.

This was the nucleus of the team that I came to rely on for management, operational success, personal trust, and just the general enjoyment of coming into the office every day. That last part actually extended to everyone at our company. The truth is that when I reflect on those days, I realize that I was assembling a family, of sorts—perhaps the one I had always wanted.

During my three years at college, each break I would come home and help coach the high school wrestling team. Still there was my old coach, whom I always referred to as Coach Chang. For some reason, I just loved to say both words in conjunction; it just has a nice ring, "Coach Chang." Anyway, he had coached me from the eighth grade all the way through high school, and he was doing the same thing for a new generation of local kids. When I returned to Martinsville from Longwood and began working at Fieldcrest Mills, I would come to the gymnasium after my shift to assist Coach Chang or work out myself. By that time, Coach Chang had hired his son-in-law, named Chad, to train as his replacement. I soon learned that Coach Chang had been diagnosed with terminal cancer, and it was not known how much time he had left to live. Chad would go on to make me assistant coach of the high school team for five hundred bucks; I was honored to accept his offer and have one more opportunity to make my Coach Chang proud.

I learned a lot of what I know today about coaching from Coach Chang and from that time spent coaching kids who were enduring a place and circumstances similar to my own when I had begun wrestling under Coach Chang's tutelage. He had told us repeatedly, like a mantra, "You don't need to know every move to win. You simply need to perfect three moves." That was his philosophy; he was a believer in the underdog. I gravitated toward that attitude. I appreciated having someone believe in me, and I brought that same philosophy from Coach Chang to my office team. Despite our underdog makeup, we would be the absolute best at a specific number of critical things, and that would become something of an unofficial motto in our office.

In Coach Chang's final years, a man who had been six foot two and roughly three hundred pounds, sporting a mustache and a mullet with spiky, gelled hair, was now weighing in at less than one hundred and fifty pounds while still wearing the same clothes. He looked like he was drowning in fabric, and yet he still came to every tournament embodying the same passion for the sport that he had always had. He was as fearless as he always had been. He had been the underdog his whole life, yet he never caved to anyone or anything. He was a pillar for all of us to gather around and seek shelter. We were all much less intimidated or nervous at away matches knowing that Coach Chang was *our* coach. A towering power was in *our* corner. What was there to fear?

In the end, Coach Chang did not surrender quietly. He did not hide. He didn't even change his clothes. He would be remembered as he was, as he always had been to us. Our coach, the giant superman forever in our corner.

I guess, in hindsight, I wanted to be something like that for my team. They were my family, and I wanted all of us be successful together. I built an environment in which the goal wasn't to accomplish through an individual's performance but rather from a culture focused on supporting and synergizing the group. Leading performers were recognized and called to share their wisdom with other team members.

Together, we were able to grow our office. Our focus was to be transparent in communication, listen to one another, and challenge one another to become a higher standard of colleagues. We applied a version of Coach Chang's strategy: Everyone doesn't need to be good at everything in order to be successful. Everyone needs to perfect their own skills, allowing us to synergize our workflow, creating a successful process and culture that wins together.

We managed to do that, and from 2007 to 2016, I was living what I thought was my best life. I was in great physical condition. My career was excelling beyond my wildest hopes. I had successfully built an office family that felt unstoppable. It was also a time of many personal and professional accolades for me.

My team and I put together the infrastructure of the company by building a new management platform, which helped grow and optimize our business exponentially. I designed and managed teams to build a purchase order management system as well as a contract management system. We continued to grow quickly. To balance the fast-paced growth, I initially led each department or initiative until I could find someone who I trusted to do it better than me, and then I would hand it over to them. I took pride in that, and I felt that not only would the entire organization be better off for it but each team member would be as well. This included imports, exports, customs brokerage, IT, onboarding, and trade compliance.

Where there is victory, however, there is also loss. All the time and energy I was putting in at the office was time and energy I could not give to anyone else, most notably Julie and Lucy. And while I was elated and energized by the success we were having at work, I was physically draining myself to the point of it being unhealthy. As is often said, nothing gold can stay.

CHAPTER SIX

CLEAR RESULTS, UNCLEAR ACTION

2017–2018

A lifeline came amid my body's deepening mysteries in 2017. The first person I confided in at the company about my diagnosis was my friend Lionel, and he agreed to keep it a secret until I was ready to announce my new reality to the others. Unbeknownst to me, Lionel thankfully broke this agreement and decided to share the news with one of our trusted colleagues, who also happened to be our company's chief legal counsel. Out of the blue one afternoon, Lionel's friend called me from the corporate office. As though an unspoken prayer had been answered, he told me that he happened to live down the street from a pretty prominent figure in the MS community, who had something to do with the MS Institute, the leading national organization on MS research. "I know he's so involved in the field that he probably has limited time to see new patients, but would you like me to ask him if he could see you?" he asked. I was floored. I hadn't heard of such an institute and hadn't yet thought to seek out such a prominent expert on the disease. "Yes, please. I would really appreciate that."

By the end of that November, I found myself face-to-face with literally one of the faces of MS-related research in America—who was not at all what I expected. He walked into the room wearing cowboy boots and blue jeans, sporting a goatee and a shell necklace, with long hair grazing his shoulders. I liked him instantly. I found relief in his willingness to listen closely to me and consider my ideas with an open mind. He didn't want to shut down any conversation; he only wanted to figure out the answers that would most help me. He explained that the cause of an MS diagnosis is extremely difficult to pinpoint, since it has origins in genetics, lifestyle, and environmental factors. He also explained that MS affects its victims individually.

Every person living with MS will experience some variation in their symptoms. The disease may impact different parts of the body at different times, progressing at different speeds and with differing levels of severity from one person to the next. He then proceeded to review the results of the new images taken earlier that morning. He explained that the images revealed I now had thirty-six lesions, spanning from my brain down my spinal cord. Nonetheless, despite hearing that the number of lesions had increased since my last scans, I felt such a relief to finally get some deeper explanations from a neurologist who seemed willing to outwork the disease that was trying hard to steal my mind and body. I went back to Martinsville reinvigorated for the fight ahead.

Work and life continued their seemingly inseparable march forward, marked by my relentless pursuit of success and control. But as the seasons changed, so did the tides of certainty. The rhythm of my usual routine started to be disrupted by subtle shifts that hinted at a future I couldn't foresee.

The echoes of my tireless dedication to work and command began to show their cracks. The random pulsing sensation in my legs that I had dismissed as a minor inconvenience took on a more frequent presence. As the months flew by in 2017, so did the unpredictability that had quietly taken root within me. Despite my determination to muscle through and attribute everything to simple overexertion, those pulses in my legs and the occasional numbness in various parts of my body had become part of my everyday life, refusing to be ignored.

For a man who prided himself on control, the lack of definitive answers with which I could develop a strategy to defend against or attack this bizarre bodily intruder was an unwelcome challenge. My usual approach of analyzing, problem-solving, and overcoming hurdles wasn't working as effectively as I'd hoped. The core of my identity was built on my being in control, and this new reality was undermining that very foundation. I had learned to maneuver through complexities and find solutions in the business world, but this was a puzzle that defied my mastery.

My other visits to medical professionals yielded only more questions. Tests came back inconclusive, leaving me with a growing sense of unease. My PCP, my confidante in physical matters, was similarly baffled. The assurance I had sought from the medical realm remained elusive, leaving a void that I struggled to fill on my own.

Amid this uncertainty, the company was similarly becoming more of a puzzle. Our efforts and innovations in the past had paid off, propelling us to new heights over the years. The fast-paced world of logistics had long provided a comforting distraction from the personal turmoil that was building within me and at home. It was a familiar realm, one where I felt most sure of myself and my role—a domain where my tenacity and control had tangible results.

For instance, unlike at our previous company, the founding members did not hold any specific titles. When Andre purchased the company in 2009, we did not have a CEO or vice president, no senior this or senior that. We all knew what one another's skill sets were and what segments of the business we were all charged with managing, but it was more unspoken than official titles on our emails or stamped onto nameplates on our office doors and desks. It was at this time that Andre created the CEO role and Lionel served as the COO while Neo and I assumed self-proclaimed titles.

We were able to maintain this cavalier approach until Andre finally sold the company to a private equity firm in 2016, whose executives required me to change my title to something with "chief" in the name. I wanted to use chief janitorial officer, but Lionel didn't think that would fly and ultimately forced me to rechoose. I finally settled on what it was that I actually did for the company and became the company's official chief solutions officer (CSO). It may seem like a minor detail, but the lack of formal titles—and the reinforcing of hierarchy that often comes with them—strengthened the feeling of family among my team in Martinsville.

I was slowly being left again, though, as Andre, Lionel, and Neo all either exited the company or tendered resignations by the end of 2017. I was the only one of our group who decided to stay, a choice that may not have sat well with everyone.

Being the only cofounder remaining, my title was once again changed to COO. This meant I was a member of the board as well as one of the "official" managers of the organization. This dual paradigm developed into me seeing myself as something of a father figure to my team, a protector, someone who owed my team the safety and opportunities most of them had never received anywhere else in their lives. I used my position to shield my team and make them as untouchable as possible so they could work in their own style and on their own terms, at least within reason. Being in the C-suite and so far from the corporate headquarters also afforded me more leeway to coach my new hires and develop them into the talent we needed. It was like finding a diamond in the rough and polishing them up, and I loved that. I had long loved to coach others, going back to my early twenties when I probably needed more coaching than anyone else.

I spent the ensuing years acting as an insulator of sorts between my team and, in my opinion, an inappropriately selected corporate management group who wanted to turn a quick profit for their investors. Their focus was on money, not what we did, meaning there was some belief that the more money we spent as a company, the larger the company would become. Now, granted, I have very limited experience at managing assets for private equity groups and working with the installation of their management hierarchies, so my commentary is within the limitations of my own paradigm, but it does suggest that this is often the case in this world. In my assessment, no one wanted to create or build value; they only wanted to use money to generate more using various ratios of spend to size. This, again, is my personal opinion based on my experiences working with five different private equity firms and many high-level executive management groups or individuals, most of whom did not have any or the right kind of supply chain experience. My frustration with their strategy was growing by the day, but I coped with that stress by focusing on my team members and making myself as helpful to them as possible.

This continued as my body, once a fortress of strength, continued to betray me. Every passing week, the sensations in my legs escalated from mere pulses to more pronounced disruptions. It became evident that this was not something I could will away with determination. The very thing I had worked so hard to master, my body, was rebelling against me.

I had built my life on controlling outcomes, so this diagnosis of a disease that no one seemed to know anything about was a seismic shift of mentality for me. It was as if the ground beneath me had crumbled, leaving me standing on shifting sands. The future, once a landscape I thought I could navigate and shape, became a nebulous expanse of wavering anxiety, hope, and bewilderment. Every plan, every aspiration, every expectation was cast into doubt.

My travel schedule was operating at a feverish pace, as my primary job throughout 2018 was to fly all over the country and beyond to evaluate opportunities, make sales calls, speak at conventions, and consult with clients to develop solutions. For example, I once flew about eight hours to Heathrow Airport in London for a three-hour meeting at the airport and then immediately jumped back on a plane and flew home. Of course, this is an example of the extreme, but these types of trips had become somewhat regular fixtures in my growing inventory of responsibilities.

The stresses of constant travel, poor access to nutritious foods, and lack of quality rest brought with them more health challenges for me. By the spring of 2018, I was taking a six-hundred-milligram cocktail of several different medications every day, all while doing my best to hide my condition from my clients and coworkers. I didn't want anyone's pity. More than anything else, I didn't want them to think I couldn't do my job. But the reality of my struggle was getting harder and harder to conceal. During one meeting with our board of directors in New York City, I felt as though my stomach had flipped and tightened like a spring. I was nauseous and knew that if I didn't leave the conference room, I would vomit everywhere. I couldn't even speak. I just silently stood up and walked out the door. I walked to a food table and began pretending to eat. I then quickly ducked around the corner to find a trash can to stand beside until the episode passed.

The constant travel had also become my paradoxical comfort zone, though. It was a way to escape the dubiety that had taken root within me, a way to distract myself from the reality of my body's growing rebellion. The airport lounges, hotel rooms, and conference halls had become my second home. In those familiar spaces, I could temporarily shelve the strangeness that lurked just beneath the surface.

But even the normalcy of routine travel couldn't shield me from the reality of my deteriorating health. The medications I was taking, the constant fatigue, and the suppressed symptoms were taking their toll. I felt like a tightly wound spring, always on the brink of unraveling. Each flight was a test of endurance, each meeting an exercise in maintaining a facade of calm and normalcy.

As my travel schedule grew increasingly demanding, the strain on my body became more evident. The once-familiar sensations in my legs had intensified, and the relentless pace of my life was charging a hefty price. My carefully constructed illusion of control was starting to crack, and it was becoming harder to hide the struggles I was facing. The daily cocktail of medications was necessary, but it was also a reminder of my vulnerability.

The incident during the board meeting in New York had been a wake-up call. It was a stark reminder that I couldn't keep pushing myself to the brink without consequences. The fear of collapsing, of being exposed, began to overshadow my every move. I realized that I couldn't keep up the charade forever, but I was going to try to do just that for as long as possible. Change wasn't something that came naturally to me. I was wired to control, to power through, to find solutions and strength in chaos. Admitting that I needed help was the toughest pill to swallow.

I vividly remember that trip to London, too. As the plane touched down at Heathrow, I felt a wave of dizziness and nausea wash over me. My head was spinning, and the plane seemed to sway as I disembarked and tried to maintain a composed exterior. The brief meeting was a blur, a haze of trying to concentrate while battling my body's rebellion. And as I boarded the return flight, the exhaustion hit me. I closed my eyes, longing for a moment of respite, but my mind was lost in a whirlwind of anxiety and confusion.

I knew that what I was doing probably wasn't the best thing for me, but I didn't know what else to do. As far as I was concerned, I was getting away with concealing this illness. I felt that I could continue with my duties at work unnoticed, especially since my team was stepping up for me and taking on more responsibilities. I had effectively had a full-time job my entire life. Going and pushing and going was all I'd ever known, no matter what the circumstances were or how I was feeling. But for the first time in my life, I wondered how long I could keep going at that pace. I felt like I was running full speed on a treadmill that I could neither stop nor escape from, and I was beginning to stumble. Except, in my mind, behind that treadmill was a bottomless pit full of unknown consequences.

By this time, I had also evolved as a leader. In my younger years, I had been aggressive and impatient with people. By the end of 2018, however, I felt I had matured and grown humbler and more understanding with my team. I was forced to trust others more and delegate tasks that I had once clung to tightly. I felt like my Poppa Ralph, in a way. He was always around, and though he wasn't the person doing everything, he would always check on everyone and do anything that needed to be done. That was, more or less, my job: the experienced caretaker, looking out for everyone but himself.

CHAPTER SEVEN

YOUR BODY, THE FOREST

2018–2019

I finally got in to see the orthopedic medicine expert, Dr. Talty, in February of 2018. When she walked into the exam room, she asked me a series of general medical questions about my lifestyle routine, ailments, family medical history, etc. She had already reviewed my growing file, which by then included several test results. Then she looked me straight in the eyes and said, "I'm going to help you." I could tell right away that she was open-minded and driven. She was also the doctor who solidified in my mind that I was in a situation that may have a future, albeit one that would likely be very challenging and yet possibly not permanent. It was an extremely difficult and frightening experience but also relieving in that there was someone who seemed to be listening intently to me for the first time—someone telling me that I had a chance to get my life back. There was real hope where there hadn't been any in a long time.

She explained that her research, specializing in Lyme disease and how it can be misdiagnosed as MS, was the subject of a lot of debate within the medical community. Her career allowed her to witness many cases and work with top professionals in this field, namely Dr. Mars. Additionally, she said that her fiancé, a pediatric thoracic surgery fellow at the University of California, San Francisco, had apparently been misdiagnosed with MS and had then stopped working. For one year, her husband-to-be was forced to go on disability while he was self-administering interferon injections every other day. Dr. Talty had been an orthopedic medicine specialist in San Francisco when she began to question her fiancé's diagnosis. Embarking on a personal crusade to discover the truth first led her to Dr. Mars and his team's research. After discovering that her fiancé had a low CD57 and running an IGeneX test that came back positive, she was convinced that he had Lyme disease rather than MS. Her fiancé agreed with her findings, and he began treatment for Lyme disease.

Over the course of a few months of treatment, he had made a full recovery, she told me, only to learn that he still couldn't practice medicine because the medical board evidently remained unconvinced that he didn't have MS; the board was doubtful that his physical and cognitive abilities were as reliable as they once had been. Tragically, he later died in a car accident after beating Lyme disease. According to Dr. Talty, prior to his untimely passing, he still hadn't been able to convince his colleagues in the field to allow him to practice even general surgery, rendering him incapable of regaining his license.

Believing that I might also be exhibiting signs of Lyme disease, Dr. Talty went to work with a series of tests and interviews with me, starting from scratch to ensure she had the correct information on my condition.

The first thing she did was show me that all three of the tests I had taken in 2017 did show that I had Lyme disease. I immediately put my head down and cried. In my mind, she was telling me I was right for doubting my diagnosis, and the feelings of relief and vindication were overwhelming in that moment.

The conversation continued, however, as she informed me to think of it this way: It wasn't that I didn't have MS; it was that we might have found my catalyst. She described what MS is and how it works. Based on her conversations with Dr. Mars at the International Lyme and Associated Diseases Society conferences in 2017, she described MS as a forest fire. "The same way you can look at a forest and identify where a fire has taken place, we can look at the nervous system and identify where MS has occurred," she said. "The question we should be asking is twofold: One, what started that fire, and two, how can we prevent future fires?"

The lesions that the neurologists had found showed where the attacks occurred; however, it was still unknown how long I'd had MS. "These lesions are like the burn scars after a wildfire," she told me. "We know that you have nearly forty lesions, or 'burn scars.' We just need to look for what caused the wildfires."

She then pulled up a chair beside me, holding sheets of paper with dozens of numbers on each one. "See this?" she asked. "These are all the different biomarkers that we have for you. The CDC (Centers for Disease Control and Prevention) guidelines, which most primary care physicians use, only count a total of IgM and IgG markers to determine if the test is positive or not. This, in fact, is too strict of a measurement to accurately determine if Lyme disease is present. For example, the CDC requires more markers in order to invoke treatment. The test can easily produce a false negative but not a false positive finding. Based on your results, you have the specific bands that only appear when the spirochete that causes Lyme disease is present. These are called signature bands," she told me. "Therefore, your test is positive. You have Lyme disease, Blake."

She proceeded to explain that, since we could not determine precisely when I had contracted it, despite knowing that I had been infected for some time now, then we could not simply throw antibiotics at the situation. We must first listen to my body to determine how we could help it remove this toxin. She then sent me off to get blood work—thirty-six vials, to be precise. When I went to the hospital, the nurse came into the room and began to lay out her work area. As she did so, she looked at the order and said, "Oh my, I've never drawn this much at one time. Hold on just one minute!" She promptly left the room and returned with two other nurses. The elder, more experienced nurses had not seen that large of an order, either. However, they did not see any issue as long as I had food in my stomach to keep me from passing out. So, I went to the cafeteria and ate about twenty-five dollars' worth of heavy food. When I returned, the ladies gathered in a coordinated fashion. It was the Henry Ford assembly line for blood work. One did the extraction while the others prepped, shook, and stored the full vials.

Ultimately, the blood work came back to tell Dr. Talty that my body was riddled with all sorts of things, meaning it probably hadn't been effectively processing bacteria and other immune-related responses for many years. "We found parasites, bartonella, babesia, lots of heavy metals, cat scratch fever, and mold in your system, in addition to active Lyme disease. We need to treat each one of these in the proper order with medication and detoxing, focusing first on the mold, then the parasites and heavy metals. This should help us get your body stable enough to treat your other illnesses."

As the new year began in 2018, that fateful visit to Dr. Talty brought the first inklings of clarity. A greater understanding of the catalyst of my diagnosis emerged, one that would reshape my reality and challenge the core of my identity through its treatment plan. I knew, and was told in even more certain terminology, that this myriad of illnesses would wreak havoc on my central nervous system and cast a shadow of unreliability over every facet of my life until we stopped the wildfires and gave the forest time to heal and potentially regrow.

While Dr. Talty's expertise and determination were comforting, her diagnosis effectively summoned God's presence on this journey in a way that I hadn't yet recognized. Whether I wanted to accept it or not, the physical, emotional, and spiritual elements of my life were colliding.

I was still trudging along at a fast pace, believing that I could outwork the questions accumulating at the company and in my body. But God had other plans. I was forced to confront my own shortcomings, not just in my work but as a human being.

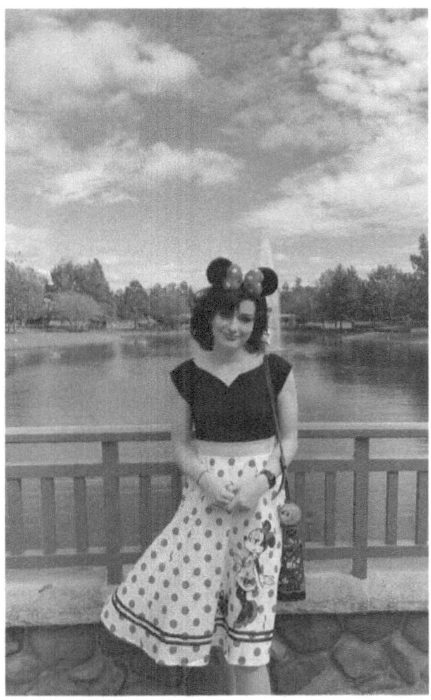

Meanwhile, as life continued to evolve around me, Lucy was growing up in the blink of an eye. As I grappled with my internal struggles, I realized that the same dedication to control that had propelled my business success was distancing me from the moments that truly mattered. Time with Lucy and Julie was slipping through my fingers like sand, and I was left with a gnawing fear that I had prioritized the wrong things.

With my team covering more duties for me at the office, I decided to take Julie and Lucy on as many trips with me as I could, including New York, Washington, D.C., Disneyworld, and elsewhere. But when their company felt distant to me, as though they were ungrateful for my presence, I was offended. Oh, the ego. "Why aren't y'all happy?" I asked angrily. "Aren't you glad I'm here, that we're all here going to these amazing places together?" To this, some equivalent of a shrug or "meh" was shot my way. It would take a few years for me to realize that I had a penance to pay for my years-long emotional absence from their lives; the road to repairing these relationships would be long and was only just beginning.

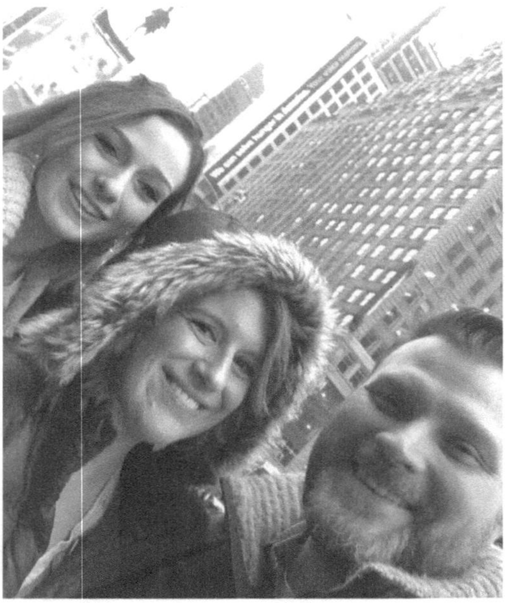

I found myself at a crossroads—faced with a choice. I could continue to fight against the current, clinging desperately to the illusion of control while trying to deceive myself and everyone around me into believing that I was fine. Or I could learn to adapt, to find strength in vulnerability, and to redefine my sense of self. It was a process of unlearning and relearning, of shedding the armor of control and allowing myself to be shaped by circumstances beyond my grasp.

The journey would be far from easy. It would demand introspection, humility, and a willingness to confront the unknown with an open heart. I would have to dismantle the walls I had built around myself and allow new and scary connections with others to form. I would have to embrace the messy, beautiful unpredictability of life. Worst of all, I would have to accept the fragility and imperfections of my own self. And I just wasn't ready for that—not yet. So, I convinced myself that I could keep up the facade of my old self: the workaholic, fix-anything, beat-anything champion of my own fate.

Then came a meeting in Houston around the summer of 2019. In the middle of a presentation, I collapsed in front of my client. She and my coworker had to rush me to a hospital in her car, occasionally stopping so I could vomit.

On the flight home, as I stared out at the patchwork of clouds beneath me, a profound realization struck me: I was living my life as though it were a linear path, a straight road with a clear destination. But the reality was far more complex, akin to a forest with winding trails, hidden clearings, and unexpected obstacles. Just as a forest is influenced by countless factors—from the weather to the soil to the creatures that inhabit it—my life was shaped by forces just as unpredictable and uncontrollable.

In that moment of clarity, I saw that I had been striving to bend the forest of my life to my will, hacking away at its branches and undergrowth to create a path of my choosing. I didn't quite understand it yet, but God was fighting back against that idea, reminding me that I was a part of something greater, something intricate and unpredictable. I couldn't control every twist and turn, nor could I predict every outcome.

As the plane touched down back home, I realized that I would have to approach my life with a new perspective. The relentless pursuit of control had led me to this point of physical and emotional exhaustion. It was time to step back and find a way to live in harmony with the forest around me, to accept that the path might not always be clear and that was OK.

Over the next few months, I began to make small changes. I started prioritizing my health, seeking out better ways to manage my condition. I opened up to my colleagues and clients about my struggles, and, to my surprise, they were supportive and understanding. I no longer saw vulnerability as a weakness but as a strength, a way to connect with others on a deeper level.

I also began to reevaluate my priorities. The fast-paced world of business was still important, but it was no longer my sole focus. Recognizing my faults wasn't enough; I would have to work on reprogramming myself. I embarked on a journey of self-discovery, seeking to understand the intricate nuances of human interaction, empathy, and communication that had evaded me my entire life. It was a humbling process, requiring me to set aside my ego and embrace vulnerability.

I started spending more quality time with Lucy and Julie. I embraced the joy of being present, *really* present, whether it was in the mundane moments or the special occasions.

As the months rolled on in 2019, my role at work evolved as well. The company began losing value as the management group continued to dedicate the firm's resources to wasteful spending and marketing to areas other than operations, and I realized that my worth wasn't solely tied to my ability to excel at every aspect of the business. It was tied to my vision, my leadership, and my willingness to learn and adapt. I would need those skills, as I could see that the end was near for the company's current management team.

Lucy, now a young woman, continued to be a beacon of light in my life as well. Our relationship was just beginning to transform from one of distance to one of deeper connection. I had learned that being present and engaged with my loved ones was far more valuable than any boardroom victory. The regrets that had once gnawed at me were replaced with a growing sense of fulfillment and gratitude.

The path ahead was still uncertain, but I was learning to embrace the uncertainty. Life was no longer a puzzle to be solved but a journey to be experienced. My body was no longer a fortress of control but a vessel for growth and transformation.

Thus far, 2019 was proving to be a year of unraveling, of shedding old skins, of gaining some medical answers but even more questions, and a new path for the company was on the horizon. The future remained uncertain, but the difference was that I was starting to understand that I wouldn't be able to control the outcomes as well as I once had. I would have to learn to dance with the future, to find joy and purpose in each step, no matter where it led. In hindsight, I believe I was just beginning to see that uncertainty, far from being a threat, was an invitation to embrace God's plan for my life in all of its unknowable glory.

CHAPTER EIGHT
PUTTING OUT FIRES

2010

It was a Sunday in early September when I got the phone call. The sky was clear, the air still and warm. And that morning I had no idea that I would never be whole again.

I answered my phone as I drove. My dad's voice sounded devastated, angry, and frightened all at the same time, unlike anything I'd ever heard from his mouth before. "Everyone says they cannot get a hold of you. Why are you not answering your phone, son? Where have you been?" he asked.

"Uh, I'm just driving around, and I don't know what you are talking about. I don't have any missed calls? Dad, what's wrong?"

"You need to get to the hospital *now*."

The call ended, and my mind began to race with scenarios of one tragedy or another. When I got to the hospital waiting room, I opened the door expecting to see my dad, but I was shocked to see the room filled with my mom's family. I'm not sure which direction he came from, but my dad walked to me and wrapped his arms around me as I made my way through the door into the middle of the room. "She's gone, son. Crystal's gone." I felt the weight of his body fold into me. I held him as he sobbed, wetting the fabric around my shoulder and chest. I didn't want to let go of him, but after several minutes, he took a deep breath, wiped his eyes with his sleeve, and gently pushed me away. "Go hug your mama," he said. "She's hurting. Go hug her."

As he pushed me toward Mom, Uncle Mike intercepted me. "Your mother is hurting and you need to go see her now, but I want you to know I love you and God loves you. Now go." Mike then continued to push me to keep me in the state of motion in which he found me.

I walked over to my mom. There she was, sitting and rocking her body side to side next to her parents, Loraine and Ralph Jarrett. I can remember Poppa nodding to me as I knelt and held Mom where she sat staring blankly at me as though she was lost in disbelief. Holding her felt different from holding my dad. There was little feeling coming from her, like she was numb. She loosely put an arm around me, swiftly and softly patting my back. I'm sure the shock of losing Crystal was weighing heavily on her, and the exchange felt empty or lifeless to me at the time.

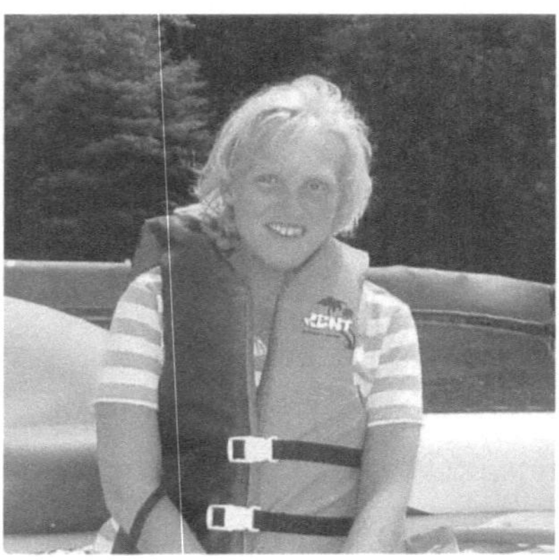

I hadn't spent much time with Crystal or Mom in the years prior to Crystal's passing. I had allowed a disagreement I had with my mother's approach to managing Crystal become a wedge in our relationship. I felt that she would rather let Crystal behave however she wanted to than use the energy to create some structure and boundaries for Crystal's life. Things had come to a head one afternoon when Lucy was still a toddler.

My mother's side of the family wanted to meet at the local Pizza Hut for lunch one weekend to celebrate my sister's birthday, so Julie and I agreed to join them. Crystal arrived in a Tigger nightgown and Winnie-the-Pooh slippers, with half her hair in a ponytail and the other half down and juice stains lining the corners of her mouth. While in line at the salad bar, a woman slightly bumped into Crystal or asked her for some space—some minor infraction of the sort. In retaliation, Crystal reared back and slapped the woman clean across her face. "Crystal!" Poppa Ralph cried out, appalled at her behavior. My mother also yelled out Crystal's name, but it appeared it was more so to cover her burst of laughter, amused at the absurdity of the scene. This was one of the first times Julie was exposed to Crystal in a public setting. The incident left her horrified and uncomfortable, wondering if we should continue to expose Lucy to Crystal, which was completely understandable after what she had just witnessed.

Tensions between my mother and me also escalated as I would either voice or harbor my concerns about how she was caring for Crystal. I knew Crystal would behave in certain ways or do the things you wanted her to do if you made her. If you did not, then she would literally do whatever she wanted to do. It was somewhere around this time that the local schools no longer allowed Crystal to attend, as she had aged out of their special needs programs. As a result, Crystal spent most of her days at home playing games and swimming. Between my contemptuous feelings toward my mother and seeing how good a man her new husband, Jim, truly was by witnessing his care and attention for Crystal, I began to myopically distance myself and focus on my career and family. At the time, I believed this distance would make everything easier for everyone.

Crystal died in her favorite place to be. She was swimming in the pool on a sunny Sunday afternoon when she suffered a heart aneurysm. She died instantly, feeling little more than a brief jolt amid the cool water and warm air. At her funeral, Uncle Mike and I filled the church with balloons for her. Her favorite cartoon was Winnie-the-Pooh (her favorite character being Tigger), and everyone brought stuffed animals, balloons, and toys featuring various characters from the series. Her funeral felt more like a child's birthday party than a burial for the dead. I'm sure it was just as she would have wanted it; after all, church was her second favorite place to be.

For the next several days, I went to my mother's house every day and spent hours talking with her. She was more verbal than she had ever been and often shared fond stories about the things I had missed with Crystal and Jim. She talked positively about God and family. It was a new version of Tammy I had never seen before, and I watched her with skepticism. I was waiting for her to show me who I had always seen when company left and the door closed. I didn't believe that she could have changed so much, so I kept believing that she was putting on a show for me and everyone else. But she never confirmed any of those assumptions to me. For nearly fifteen years now, she has remained this way—a kinder, more loving person. I think between Jim, her recommitment to Christ, and the loss of Crystal, something changed within her. I give the glory to God that she is a softer person than she was when I was under her care.

Crystal's death marked a profound change deep within me. I held some guilt over not spending as much time looking after her in the years leading up to her death. She was a major part of my life for such a long time. It was not easy to think about how she might have viewed my behavior—or rather, my disappearance—and how those decisions changed her perception of me, her big brother who for so long had always been with her.

2019

For the first couple years after my initial MS diagnosis, I believed I would find a way to beat it. I could often convince myself that the disease would pass, that everything would soon return to normal. By 2019, though, I was feeling worse physically and mentally. I was spending more time in hospitals, labs, and doctors' offices, and it was dawning on me that this new reality in my life wasn't going away.

As the months went by, I continued to travel and work, hoping that it would distract me from my new reality. So much was changing within me that I wanted to hold tightly to anything familiar and routine. I craved normalcy and work gave me at least some semblance of that.

After that fateful trip to Houston when my client had to rush me to a hospital in the summer of 2019, it began to dawn on me how serious my condition really was and that my life may forever be changed. Shortly before I went to Houston, I learned that the CEO (Eric) hired by the private equity group was allegedly planning to replace me as COO. As you can imagine, that news didn't invoke any comfortability with slowing down. And I certainly didn't welcome the idea of informing him that I had been diagnosed with a disease that would likely hinder, to unknown degrees, my physical and mental capabilities over time. I began pretending that I was fine so often that I almost came to believe that I was. It was different from denial, though. I felt that I needed to hide what was happening to me from so many people that, in doing so, I subconsciously thought there really was nothing wrong.

Though I hadn't wanted to tell Eric about my health issues because I feared he would fire me, after the Houston trip, I felt that I didn't have much of a choice. Immediately following the debacle in Houston, I flew to the corporate office without the intention of telling him about my diagnosis.

Eric had been installed as CEO mostly due to his career working in high-profile corporate positions. He was a very successful individual and leader, more so experienced with bureaucratic positions within the world of ground networks or marine terminals. This was his first experience within the world of an NVOCC specializing in international ocean and air freight management and solution development. Additionally, I would be remiss if I didn't say he was one of the most charismatic people I've ever met in my life. Seriously, he was a super nice guy who could get along with anyone, and he genuinely enjoyed playing the role of a leader or the patriarch. He was good at it, too. He had a clear system for this type of cultural development.

Although I rarely agreed with his choices of direction to drive our organization, I decided to listen and compromise with the goal of understanding why those choices were being made. This proved to be a valuable lesson for me, as Eric helped me learn how to apply what I call the "Andre style" of business in new ways, which was to sell the potential of what an idea could be. Eric's approach was a more polished corporate view, in which ideas are expressed with a jargon and collateral more suitable to bankers and private equity groups. At the end of the day, I could see his strengths and worked on learning those skills from him.

During my visit to the main office, Eric and I went to eat lunch at the food court in one of the local malls, and as we were riding down the escalator back to the office, I completely lost my train of thought mid-sentence. I felt like I was in space—you know, based on the idea that nothing happens in the way you are used to it happening. I was also completely unaware of anything that had happened that day prior to this strange moment. *What did I just say?* I thought to myself. *What's happening? What are we talking about?* I started to panic. It was probably the most scared I have ever felt in a single moment because, in my mind, I knew right then and there that I was becoming an invalid. My immediate thought was that I was about to be useless, and that frightened me more than anything ever had before.

I stood there, frozen, searching for my words until Eric spoke. "Oh, don't worry about it, son. You think probably twenty times faster than the average person. The fact that you understand and can do the things you talk about is amazing to me." Eric was so compassionate in a fatherly kind of way that I let down my guard.

I thought I had played it off, but internally, I was so terrified that it must have shown outwardly to Eric. The entire walk back to the office, I tried to remember what we had been meeting about and discussing all morning, let alone what we had just been talking about in the plaza. When we got back to his office, I told him the truth. "Eric, I want you to know that I have MS." Again, Eric surprised me with his empathy, even getting vulnerable with me. He proceeded to explain his wife's health challenges and offered me tips, such as how pumpkin seeds help detox your body. The conversation was so supportive that I took the opportunity to confront Eric about the rumors of him wanting to replace me as COO. Eric proceeded to assure me that any such things were not true and that if he were to ever think about repositioning me, he would talk to me both directly and first.

The meeting offered some reprieve from my worries, but something still felt wrong to me—a feeling of concern that I couldn't quite pinpoint. I knew that my job, like most, was never completely safe, but I also believed I should be more relieved than I was. The way I have always approached everything is that, as long as I can think about it, I'm less afraid of it happening. Now I knew that my memory and ability to focus my thoughts were being taken away from me, and that was scary.

Those fears were compounded by even more uncertainty in the early fall of 2019, when Eric informed the executive team that the private equity firm wanted to start doing some prep work to sell the company. Immediately before this bombshell announcement, Eric had hired a consultant named Mark—a brilliant strategist who had been working with our company for the previous ten months—into a newly created position: chief global forwarding officer and head of third-party logistics services. Essentially, I viewed this decision as being made to replace me as COO by creating a new position to split responsibilities, with my title being changed back to CSO but with the added role of serving as the head of fourth-party logistics services. With this change, Eric eliminated the COO position altogether. At the time, Eric's words that the private equity firm wanted him to sell the company seemed more speculative than anything else, as though he wanted to keep the management of the sale to himself rather than communicate any direct statements from our private equity partners or reveal any specific definitive plans. Nonetheless, this was unknowingly one of the few times we actually received some information regarding the process. The outlook wasn't good, yet I was able to find an ally in Mark.

I cannot remember exactly when it happened, but shortly after his announcement, Eric and I had a conversation about the nature of his management changes. I asked him point-blank, "You said you would notify me of any such thoughts prior to any change; what was that?" The conversation became heated as he proceeded to explain to me that Mark's addition was not a reflection of me as COO. Rather, it was his move to creatively rebrand our services from the view of one company to the view of two revenue streams for the big sale that the ownership group was pushing toward. Despite understanding his logic, emotions were not controlled very well on either of our parts. This was the last time he and I spoke to each other one-on-one for the rest of the year. Thereafter, I decided not to be as emotional. I embraced the fact that a new ownership group would be coming in soon and looked forward to the day of the change. I continued to work closely with those who impacted the business—namely, sales, operations, and tech—to ensure that any new buyers would find value in the guts of the organization. The leaders of each respected division agreed, and together we maintained a strategy to remain unified for our customers' sake and for the sake of company performance.

One November evening after work, I sat on my porch and contemplated the future of the company and my own place in it. I was no longer on the board, so I felt completely in the dark regarding the decisions being made that would ultimately dictate all our fates. I asked God to tell me what I should do. In one of the most profound moments of my life (the kind that you don't tell anyone about and it takes things actually happening before you understand it—that type of profound), I closed my eyes, and just like I was watching a movie, I could see all the people I loved in motion. I saw my work family, my actual family, my friends. They were all real and vivid, hopeful and happy. I saw my role in their lives and how I could serve each one of them, how I must serve them. God showed me everything, telling me that, if I followed His plan, everything would happen just as it had unfolded in that movie in my mind. It seemed like a dream, but I was fully conscious and could remember every detail.

In early December, while Mark was in town working in our office, we had a closed-door meeting with just the two of us. I opened up to him about my fears and distrust of what we were not being told. He agreed and helped me focus on things we could, or rather should, control. One of his suggestions was maintaining the priority to protect everyone's jobs. To my surprise, having only recently begun feeling like I could trust Mark, he and I agreed wholeheartedly on how to set and order our priorities. We both began writing ideas as we brainstormed together on a whiteboard in my office, deciding what our game plan should be if our hunch proved to be true. We agreed to keep these conversations quiet and carried on with our day-to-day responsibilities as usual.

Weeks later, I issued to my team an "all hands on deck, go until we're done" request to process a large number of transactions we desperately needed to audit. I knew it would be a long night, and I wanted to show my appreciation to the team by ordering several boxes of pizza. Shortly into the evening, I began to feel my body seizing up, a now-familiar numbness overtaking me. It was seven thirty in the evening, and we were nowhere close to being finished, yet I knew something was off, as though I was shutting down. Not wanting anyone to see me like that, I sent everyone home and went into my office, closing the door behind me.

Within minutes, I collapsed on the floor. I struggled to fish my phone out of my pocket. When I finally retrieved it, I called Julie and mumbled, "I need you to come … get me … office." She immediately called my dad, and together they rushed to my side. They were both in shock upon their arrival and called 911 for an ambulance, which whisked me away for yet another hospital visit.

While lying in my hospital bed, a nurse repeatedly told me, "It must've been all that pizza you ate." In pain and becoming increasingly frustrated with finding so few medical professionals willing to listen to me, I took hold of her sleeve and said, "It's not the damn pizza. I never said I ate the pizza. Do you hear me?"

I was ultimately cleared to go home after a few hours, but the experience solidified in my mind, and in the minds of my family, that I was entering a new phase of vulnerability and could not continue pushing myself as hard as I had been for so many years. A new beginning was ahead of all of us, and the uncertainty of what that would look like left us embroiled in fear and anticipation.

CHAPTER NINE

A NEW (BEE)GINNING

2020

From the very start of 2020, I began accepting my newfound physical limitations. I knew I couldn't hide my condition from everyone much longer, so instead I set out to find ways that I could still be useful and productive. The year would begin, however, with yet another difficult loss when Poppa Ralph died on the second Monday in February.

In some ways, his death—and the inevitable pull back to my extended family that came with it—compelled me to push even further into my career. I wanted to distract myself from my familial grief and pain and memories. The fear of going backward in any way terrified me at the time. It felt like my own bodily future was being stolen from me, and the only area of my life that I had any control over was my work. I found solace there. I found purpose there. I found my strength and usefulness there—all things that I felt I had lost and may never find again. I had a new North Star, so I could forget about the problems I needed to face. At the time, it sounded like the perfect plan: Ignore my own pain and battles; fight everyone else's instead.

While Eric had initially told us back in August of 2019 that he had been ordered to sell the company, the private equity team had already cut its funding to the company. It was essentially going to let it die on the vine unless someone could find a buyer. In the first week of January in 2020, Eric came to Mark and me and explained what was happening. He proceeded to describe the next steps. Since no buyer could be found and the bank would likely put the assets up for sale, we would have a chance to purchase certain assets ourselves.

"The ownership group has been trying to find a buyer for months, but no one's made a bid. If there are no bidders within the next week or so, the bank will likely put the company into foreclosure. If that were to happen, they'll break the company down and sell it for parts. It's small, but this could present an opportunity for us to potentially rebuild a company from scratch. We could probably pick up the intellectual property—the system that you built, Blake—for about five hundred thousand. Now, I'm good for three hundred grand. I could probably do more, but I wanted to talk to you and Mark and see if you guys want to come in on it with me."

I was incensed that Eric had withheld this knowledge from us for four or five months and now wanted us to sit back, let people lose their jobs, and then try to pick up the pieces for our personal benefit, all in less than two weeks.

"Somebody could submit a bid in two weeks, Eric."

"Maybe, but at this point, that is highly unlikely ..." he told me.

The next day, Eric, Mark, and I had a conference call with another executive member, who had undesirably decided to join in Eric's idea to build a new company in the event of foreclosure. Mark and I knew that neither of them knew much about our industry—or the business itself, really. Frankly, I did not want to be part of a new company with co-owners who would inevitably make bad decisions on behalf of the management group, the employees, and our customers. The company's financial performance since the purchase provided enough evidence that I needed to find another way to save the company.

The day after that phone call, I swallowed my pride, compiled a presentation, and drove to the office of an old high school classmate, Jesse H. Wade III, who was now running a very successful financial investment and wealth management firm in town. Jess and I had something of a one-sided rivalry in high school. The son of a former CFL and NFL quarterback, he was muscular and athletic without having to try very hard to be either. He and his family lived on the "good" side of town with all the other "good" kids who wore expensive clothes, drove nice cars, and sported Ivy League haircuts. Sometimes, you instinctively don't like someone simply because you assume they won't like you. That was our dynamic, even though I think Jess was completely unaware that such an arrangement existed in my mind.

While I spent most of my time trying to improve my wrestling, Jess, a starter on the football team who would receive college scholarships for his skills, wasn't too interested in enhancing his athletic gifts. He had everything I had ever dreamed of, and yet his only concern was getting out of school. I was envious, and I'd always assumed that Jess knew that. I'd also guessed that he might have enjoyed knowing that I envied him. I was wrong on both accounts. But on that afternoon, some twenty-odd years later, when I was standing outside his building, I still felt like that shaggy kid from Clearview/Jones Creek crawling across the tracks to ask a favor of the popular jock who had it all.

I was trembling with nerves and anticipation when I knocked on the door. To my surprise, despite having a secretary and other people working for him in the front, Jess opened the door himself and looked down at me from the stoop. Though we hadn't seen each other since high school, he recognized me immediately. "Blake! Hey, buddy!" he said, smiling. I replied, "Hey, Jess. How are you doing?"

He shook my hand firmly and invited me into his office. Sitting across from him at his desk, I gave him my elevator pitch for why buying our company would be a good investment. He leaned back in his leather Hancock and Moore chair, fidgeting with a Montblanc pen in his hand, his jaw slightly open. He stared at me for a few seconds, during which it seemed as though time itself had stopped altogether. Then he sat up and said, "I'm not going to buy the company, but I'll help *you* buy it."

The moment he said those words, my heart stopped. All the nervousness and jitters went away. I remembered the movie in my mind, and, as it played, I could see all the people I knew who could help me. I thought of the capital opportunities available to us—all the people I could get in front of and what I could say to them. I could spit out enterprise values, current and potential partnerships and beneficial relationships, and so on. Excitedly, I unloaded all of this detailed information onto Jess. He looked baffled, presumably impressed that I knew as much as I did about business in general and the ins and outs of the company and the supply chain industry. Just as excitedly, he said back to me, "I can get you in front of as many private equity groups as you like. This is more than doable, and I would be glad to work with you on this. Let's do it!"

It was like my prayers from that fateful November evening were beginning to be answered; the movie was becoming real. I couldn't believe it. And then a tornado of missteps and deception began to form in the figurative blue skies above.

Eric was in Los Angeles when I called him the following day. "I'm going to purchase the company," I told him. "That's great, Blake. I know we are," he said. I wanted to be honest with him. "No, Eric, I don't think I'm being clear. We are not buying parts of the company. *I* am going to put in a bid to buy the entire company, and there may be others to pull onto the team, but, Eric, I'm afraid you aren't going to be one of them. I can't have you as a co-owner. I'm sorry. I don't want you to take this the wrong way. It's not that I don't like to work with you. I've come to appreciate working with you. In fact, I've learned so much from you. But, Eric, I honestly think you're best in two scenarios: in front of bankers and in front of investment groups. That's it. If you were willing to do those things as an investor or board member, and if the right people were running the company, we would all be amazing together because you're one of the best I've ever seen in front of those audiences."

You may be able to guess how the conversation went from there. Eric was livid. He couldn't believe that I, who had always seemed to be his non-adversarial and submissive sidekick, was planning to take over what he believed to be his company and then demote or fire him. Eric told me that I was making a mistake and that we would see about my plans, suggesting his own intent to buy the company or at least derail my purchase of it.

With Jess's introduction, I hired an investment firm out of New York with a large portfolio to put together a bid for me as fast as possible. The goal was to place and win the final bid, being accepted by the bank with as many equity partners as we could find. The assumption was that, if I won the bid and had multiple funding options to choose from to finance the purchase, then we could strike a deal with whichever one wanted the least to do with operating the business.

I shared with Jess one of the ideas from Mark's and my whiteboard session, which was to win the bid and then, hopefully, convince Andre to come in and help buy the business back with me or just let him take the lead. That was my ideal outcome: getting the team back together. Once I had become the last founding member left at the company, all the high-level conversations were about "keeping an eye on Andre" or rumblings of similar distractions. I never bothered to figure out what was true or what was not; I simply made sure to never reach out to anyone. I had the discipline, and I knew that was the best decision for both myself and the group—no matter how much I missed speaking with them. As a result, I had not spoken to any of them in years. Buying the company was my idea of a supreme family reunion; it was not just an opportunity to save everyone's job but a real chance to right the ship.

I received the New York firm's confidence rating; they whipped up a portfolio of three backers based on my requirements for operational funding and involvement. Choosing one of the letters of support provided, I chose to submit knowing that more options were coming as planned. Then, suddenly, the bank notified us that they were stopping the bidding process. "We're going to delay it one day," their representatives told us. "There's someone that we're going to allow to place a bid, so we're going to give them the time to do that." This was extremely peculiar, especially since there were already two other unexpected parties participating in the bid, and I instantly felt my stomach twist into a knot. Something was wrong. Something bad was going to happen. I could feel it.

Twenty-four hours later, I learned that the mystery bidder was Andre himself. Immediately, I called his attorney and asked him to arrange a call between us on his line. "I just learned that he's putting in a bid. I was told he would not be permitted. I need to talk to him," I told the attorney. He quickly arranged the call, and Andre and I jumped on the line. Andre asked questions, and I gave him honest answers about where his bid needed to be I was one hundred percent comfortable with him winning.

"What are you doing?" Andre asked, and I told him my number.

"You went that high?"

"Andre, that will win the bid."

"I don't think it's worth that much."

Andre hung up and bid just under my number. Not surprisingly, my bid was accepted. Against all odds, I won the auction to buy the company that I had helped build, when just hours earlier, I had thought it would be lost forever. Everyone was calling to congratulate me; old acquaintances, friends, and more were coming out of the woodwork. My old friend Gene heard the news and called to tell me how proud he was of me; I nearly wept over that one.

Even Andre called me afterward. "It's done. Congratulations, Blake. You got it," he told me.

"Well, I still want to work together," I said. "My hope was if I bought the company … Andre, my whole goal is for us to find a way to work together again. My plan is to come down there and see if you guys really want to buy it or just come in on it with me."

"Wait a minute, wait a minute. So you're doing all this just to get me involved?"

"Yeah. I want to get the company back to the way it was. It was perfect then, and I believe we can do it again."

"Interesting," Andre said. I could tell from his tone that he didn't believe me.

Nevertheless, I began doing the work to finish the deal. As it turned out, I was completely wrong in thinking that if I had multiple investors, then I could simply change from one to the next on my list in the event one stalled or failed to close. The bankers would only talk to whichever private equity group or investor I listed on my letter of intent. That was my downfall. The group that I had initially listed was in the middle of a massive real estate transaction and could not give me the capital until that deal closed. I was locked in and unable to change to another source. What made matters worse was that, since our funding had been cut back in August, the company was operating on cash flow, and the clock to find new capital was ticking. After three weeks of waiting, I grew impatient and decided to go back to the bank, explain the situation, and tell them that I wanted to change my lead investor out with another one on my list in order to close sooner. Then came the lawyers. By trying to make a source change, I would essentially be defaulting on my bid. In the eyes of financial law, I had submitted a fraudulent letter of intent, so I was forced to withdraw it to avoid getting sued.

After releasing control, the drama continued through two more rounds of bidding, with the next winner also being forced to release control. In the end, the banks put the company into bankruptcy, and, by way of auction, Andre became the owner of select assets, including all of the employees, for a second time. He ultimately restructured those assets into a completely new entity. I traveled shortly thereafter to meet with Andre and Lionel. It was not exactly a warm reunion, at least in my mind. They still seemed to see me as a competitor at best, and a traitor at worst. By the time I left that meeting, I had the sense that I would not remain a part of my work family for much longer. I felt like I had been standing on a frozen, crackling lake for nearly a year, and now a heatwave was coming to finish the job. Yet, I was still committed to the goals Mark and I had set back in December to support and save as many jobs as possible.

Coincidently, in late spring of 2020, Lionel called to tell me that they wanted to downsize and move our Martinsville offices into a smaller space. "Do it quietly, though," he said. For weeks, my team and I spent nights and weekends moving furniture, computers, files, and other equipment to a few different locations.

The few hours that I was home, I could tell that Julie and Lucy didn't really want to be around me. I had pushed everyone away and become someone I didn't want to be, even though I believed I had done it all with good intentions. In a game of lies and deception, sometimes it's costly to tell the truth.

Throughout that summer, Andre and Lionel didn't want me to do anything, so I began a tedious waiting game. As that old expression goes, "Idle hands are the devil's workshop." I became weak and fearful during that period of uncertainty and boredom. For the first time since my diagnosis, I truly felt my body. I could feel everything—how frail I had become, how unstable and tired I was. It was at this time that I realized I had inadvertently lost more than eighty-five pounds since my ER visit the previous December. I had not understood it before because I had blinders on for the sake of my work and my team, but now those aspects of my life were slipping through my fingers. There were no more distractions, nowhere else I could hide from the things I didn't want to admit were serious and real and unending. I couldn't understand my pain before, but I could understand it then because I was being forced to sit and feel it. I spent my days sitting at home alone, knowing I was no longer the person I had been imagining myself to be. And worst of all, I was the one who had done it to myself. I knew every step taken, every decision that I could have changed. We all know our mistakes at one time or another in our lives. Everything we do, the good and the bad, is who we are. Learning to accept that person and improve is the only way, I believe, that you can find any peace within yourself.

I made the decision to resign and take care of myself. *Let them do what they want to do*, I said to myself. *I don't need to fight anymore.*

After that choice, I found comfort—a calm that I hadn't felt in years, if ever. I wanted to rebuild my family, reconnect with God, and start healing myself. So, that's what I set out to do.

*

The forest of life continued to surprise me, but instead of resisting the unseeable horizons, I learned to let God guide me, to adapt and ride through His landscape without being in control. I surrendered to the unknown, to my limitations, and put my faith in God's vision for me. And in doing so, I found a sense of peace and fulfillment that I had never experienced before that summer.

Looking back on those years with the NEWCO and the years immediately after my diagnosis, I am grateful for the challenges and uncertainties that reshaped my life. MS was not the enemy I had feared, but rather, it could be a catalyst for growth and transformation. The forest of life is vast and unknowable, but there is beauty in the unexpected. I wanted to learn how to savor the richness of being in the present moment. The future is uncertain, which is scary, but it's also full of the potential to be greater than we expect or imagine it will be.

As the seasons shifted from summer to fall once again, so did my perspective. The relentless pursuit of success and control that had defined me for so long began to give way to a new understanding. I started to see that success wasn't measured solely by accomplishments and power but by the ability to adapt, grow, and find strength in vulnerability. My journey with MS was teaching me a different kind of strength—one that was rooted in self-awareness, resilience, and the courage to face the unknown.

With time, the rhythms of my life began to find a new balance. My body was no longer a battleground but a complex ecosystem that required care and attention. The medicines remained, but they were no longer a source of shame. They were a reminder of my journey, a testament to my willingness to embrace change and face adversity head-on. I was not done, though. God was calling me to a new beginning. He was calling me to use—really use—the knowledge, skills, and passion that had grown within me over two decades.

Maybe for the first time in my life, I didn't feel like I was in a competition. I wanted the so-called "underdogs" to win. I had felt like I was worthless my whole life, like I would never be anything special. I had won despite the odds and doubts and obstacles that for so long had riddled my path, but it took a long time for me to honestly acknowledge exactly what I had accomplished and why. God had been guiding me the whole time, even when I was sure I was completely alone. Now, I could accept that fact, and I knew that others must be feeling the same way. Only now I had the awareness that I could do something about it. Through prayer, God showed me that I am not useless. It is not about me or what I can do or even what my condition has taken from me; it is about my capacity to support and push others. Thus, the idea was born that I too could become an investor—moreover, an investor in people—to create a thriving culture. This ultimately led to two ideas to fulfill that mission. One was to create a company that uses technology and services to redesign the way supply chains are managed. The company would be called "alliancebee," which was a name that resonated as a symbol and metaphor for the teamwork, unity, trust, and work ethic that exemplified the vision. After all, what place works harder and more collaboratively than a hive of bees? Forming alliancebee was an exercise in creating a culture in which the members of my work family are listened to, encouraged, and supported so they can become the best versions of themselves, as well as treating the workplace like a mission field. And the other prong to the vision God had shown me was to create a nonprofit, community-building organization that would be called "Beegins with You." The goal behind this foundation was to not only begin living, loving, listening, and helping those in our community but also to create something with my family, Julie and Lucy.

Erecting an organization from scratch in which I could use the skills and knowledge I had gained over the years to empower others seemed like the best response to His call. This time, though, I understood what was most important. It wasn't money. It wasn't a pat on the back from the kind of people who count the pats. This time, it was about creating a work family that would live and prosper long after I was gone. This time, it was about giving opportunities to others with integrity and doing things the right way by learning to support others who do things differently than I would do them. This time, it was about building something that we could all be an equal part of. This time, it was about eternity.

CHAPTER TEN

IT BEGINS WITH YOU

2022

As I reflect on my journey, it becomes clear that my calling transcends mere professional and personal success. In the years after my medical diagnosis, a new series of challenges tore through the area of my life that I had always felt was most in my control. Suddenly, I had lost my job, my teammates, and my identity as a worker, protector, and provider. I didn't know what to do. I licked my wounds for months, wondering what I should do next, worrying if I would ever have any value to anyone again. Those months were among the darkest of my life. I had been enduring such physical and emotional turmoil for years, but in 2020, I suddenly felt that I had nothing to hang on to nor any way to offer value to Julie and Lucy. There was no place to escape to, nor did I feel there was any way to find a new purpose. I had no work family—no work at all, in fact—and the isolation and insecurity that was born from those feelings leveled me.

I began to read the Bible in a way I never had. I read it from cover to cover for the first time in my life, a truly immersive dive into the Scripture, seeking answers and guidance. Then I remembered the moment I had experienced with God on that November evening on my porch, the one during which I saw a movie that I still couldn't shake from my mind. *Everything you're doing goes against Me,* I heard within me. *Everything from now on is about service, about surrendering to your higher purpose.* I saw that same vision, but this time it was a race. It was a race that I could see I was winning. Only now, instead of racing and trying to win, I found myself going back to help others overcome their obstacles. I discovered more enjoyment not by trying to finish the race but by simply trying to help others during the race. That was the moment I realized that God wanted me to lift others up. It wasn't my place to lead. Sure, He gave me the knowledge, but now He was teaching me to discern when those things should occur and giving me the wisdom to seek His guidance to understand why they must occur.

During this time, although I was listening to God, I also began to argue with Him. This was my way of controlling how I surrendered. It was through prayer, through deep discussions with God, that I developed two mentalities. I felt that He was telling me, "Do not worry about your physical problems. Do not worry about your memory loss. If you live my way, you will never forget." To this day, God's words telling me to "live it, and you will never forget it" have been burned into my memory. Those scary moments still arrive, and they arrive more frequently than I would like. But every day, those words help me make decisions based not on what I think I know but rather on what God would have me do.

I also became very strong in the belief that I would die at the age of forty-five. As strange as it may sound, that clear timeline gave me a definitive project plan to get things done. I accepted, and I sought to bring Him glory in my final days. That belief, conviction, fear, or whatever you want to call it helped me develop an "in the moment" mentality. All of these epiphanies and changes led to my extraction out of this dark period and onto a path of service that would ultimately bring me more light and fulfillment than I had ever felt in my life.

Pulling out of the darkness through a calling to be of service is what laid the foundation for both alliancebee and Beegins with You. Through my conversations with God, I saw how my skills and experiences could be an opportunity to help everyone around me. A curse had become a blessing. I had always believed in myself and my ability to work successfully for others in whatever ways they needed me to work, but I never really had a desire to be *the* leader. Rather, I wanted to help others become leaders. I wanted to be someone else's beacon of hope, a navigator of sorts along a confusing path that can often end unexpectedly and unwantedly. With both alliancebee and Beegins with You, I wanted to invest in people and hopefully help them see what they are capable of in ways they might not have imagined previously. Particularly with our foundation, this was a way for me to invest in and lift up my family by working together and building something to serve our community.

Even so, every day, I was fighting an urge to take control of my and others' journeys. Those were the days—and I still have them even now from time to time—that I must slap myself on the wrist and say, "No. Let this go the way God wants it to go. Get out of the way." I prayed regularly for guidance and wisdom as I began this new chapter of my life, and I always heard the same answer. "You're the one who has been doing wrong. Support people, and it will heal you." I believed in it so much that I was willing to invest every ounce of energy I had into it. Quickly, I learned that, if I followed God's will rather than my own, I could find healing. The less inhibited I was while pursuing God's plan, the better I felt in the end. The whole point of that vision I had experienced on my porch that November, I later realized, was God showing me how to surrender control. And part of surrendering control required me to allow failure. I had to be willing to experience my personal sense of "failure" in order for God's plan for me to succeed. He was teaching me how to use my skills to help others instead of myself.

During this initial transition came many painful lessons of loss—loss of control, loss of loved ones, loss of a sense of my own self and power. In early 2021, two of my friends-turned-brothers, Derrick and James, were checked into the hospital. One would come out to never be the same. The other would never leave. This was a dramatic moment of failure for me because I was unavailable to help either. It was a very uncomfortable feeling. Losing our big brother James really compounded the pain and continued to push me further down a path of introspection— thoughts of all the times growing up that James had recited Scripture or explained to us *why what we were doing was a bad idea*, and just his general expression of faith that God would see us through all things. All of this happened while I was continuing to have challenges with the people I selected to run the nonprofit and for-profit organizations, both board members and employees. But God was with me through it all. He helped me understand my decisions, control my emotions, and evolve into the person He needed me to be. As painful as all those lessons were, I'm grateful for them all. The lessons continue still, through good times and bad.

Proverbs 6:6–8 says, "Go to the ant, you sluggard; consider its ways and be wise! It has no commander, no overseer or ruler, yet it stores its provisions in summer and gathers its food at harvest." I had always felt like that ant. I worked hard and had never really had a "ruler." Instead, I had been allowed to run my teams unencumbered by anyone, so long as we produced great results. I had always been the "how" guy, and throughout my career, I had always needed a "why" guy. Through God, I now had a new, more powerful "why," and I still had the know-how I'd gained over my decades of working in the supply chain industry and managing people—know-how that I could now use to execute God's plan. It made sense for me to begin investing in something to which I could lend my knowledge and as much energy as I could, while letting others elevate it to greater levels on their own.

The decision to establish a nonprofit organization stemmed from this newfound belief in the power of service and the transformative impact it can have on others. I realized that I was not alone in my struggles—that there were countless others facing their own battles, yearning for the same sense of hope and belonging I had craved throughout my life. For both Julie and me, it was a natural extension of our desire to make a tangible difference in the lives of others. It allowed us to work together and with friends and family. Julie served as the executive director of our nonprofit foundation, which led us down a path to become closer by working together.

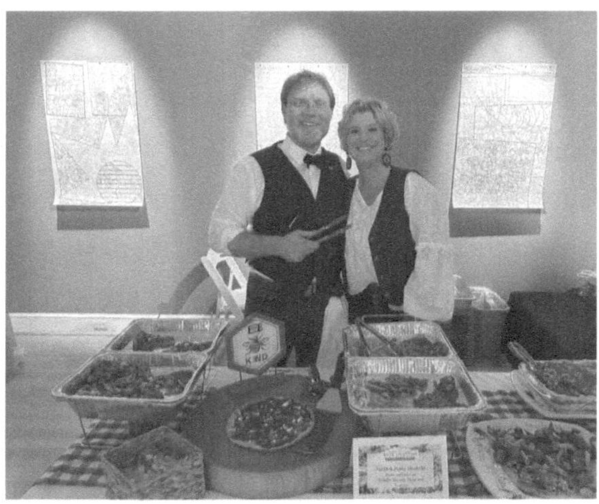

Although, the word "closer" may not be the word she would use. I drove her nuts with a triage notification system of tasks needing her attention that I would prepare for her every day. Let's just say that this methodology provided passion in our lives … maybe? In all seriousness, our relentless pushing of one another has opened so many new facets of our relationship; she is my person, on every level.

Several months later, my father—who was already peacefully retired—also came on board to serve as property manager for the building that alliancebee owns. For Dad, a relaxing way to retire is by working with his hands. Asking my father to help me afforded us an opportunity to see each other more, work alongside one another, and just enjoy the quality father–son time together that we had missed out on when I was young. I guess it makes sense that I asked him to join. When I was twenty-one years old, my father gave me the single greatest piece of advice in my life. "There are people who may not consider me a smart man," he told me, "but I didn't pay attention to that. You are what you surround yourself with, so I always try to surround myself with smart people." I have used that advice my entire career. Today, I'm not only trying to surround myself with smart people; I'm trying to immerse myself with my family as well as with the kinds of people I want to be surrounded by.

My arrangement with my father also afforded me an opportunity to potentially help him with a small strip of land that he had been taking care of for more than thirty years. Without going into detail, let's just say that I found an opportunity to help my father. I spoke with my attorney friends, found a clear-cut path, and rolled out the plan to my dad, and we proceeded to move forward. Then, out of nowhere, everything came to a halt. I wanted to keep fighting because I wanted to help my father. My dad simply looked at me and said, "Oh well, I guess the Lord doesn't want me to have it. At least not right now. Anyway, I've got to run a few errands. I'll see you tomorrow." And that was it. *How could he drop the conversation so easily?* I thought. Once again, God used that opportunity to teach me yet another lesson about surrender and listening. He was reiterating to me that I must surrender control.

*

Since its inception, the impact of the foundation has been nothing short of transformative. In addition to helping students receive care they would otherwise miss out on, our team regularly volunteers to provide essential resources to those in need. We offer services to those struggling with personal challenges, spearhead project-learning initiatives for underprivileged youth, and more. The ripple effect of our efforts knows no bounds. But beyond the tangible outcomes lies something even more profound: the restoration of faith, the rekindling of hope, and the belief that tomorrow holds promise no matter how bleak today may seem.

After a few years working as CEO of the foundation and leading its youth services program, Julie made the difficult decision to embark on her own long-standing dream of attending law school, meaning she would no longer have the time to volunteer with the kids involved in the program she had designed. We did experience a few bumps in the road trying to distribute her responsibilities among the board members, but once again, God's plan led me right to where I needed to be. Because Julie's choice to attend law school meant there was little time to wait, I stepped in to temporarily fill the role of directing our youth services division.

Back at Longwood, accounting had been my first declared major. After that first year, when I was offered a wrestling scholarship and won both individual and team accolades, I was also invited to work with Coach Chang and the kids. I decided these were all signs that I should become a coach and teacher, so I changed my major to special education. I knew I had to work within the school's system if I wanted to be a coach, and I had always been inspired by the level of impact my sister's teachers had on her life. After a probation that restricted my return to pursue that path, I began making choices to use those skills in a more selfish light—at least, that was how His Holy Spirit convincted me. The reality is that I see He was always with me, preparing me for His will.

With Julie stepping down, I found myself in a circular position of life. At the time, I did not like to work with kids, nor could I connect with them. But I didn't panic. Instead, I focused on one simple fact: This was not my plan; I must serve. I began to immediately focus on keeping everything in motion and working to figure out who should be doing this work in my stead.

To date, however, it is one of the most rewarding things I've ever done in my life. I had a chance to mentor kids, many of whom have home lives and mentalities that very much reminded me of my own at their age. To have the possibility to use what I had learned from both my childhood and my career to potentially improve their lives and their outcomes was surreal to me. The opportunity came to fruition the same way everything else has happened in my life, with God telling me, "It begins with you." I don't want anyone to feel alone, a feeling I have known too well throughout my life. For me, this duty was about showing up and being present, ensuring in the best way I could that no one in our program ever felt alone.

My own health issues have undoubtedly shaped the trajectory of this journey. They have taught me resilience in the face of adversity, humility in times of triumph, and the profound importance of empathy. Each day is a reminder that life is fragile, that every breath is a gift to be cherished. And yet, it is precisely this fragility that gives life its beauty, its urgency, and its meaning.

Those truths sound nice, but I had never been able to fully articulate how it feels to have my paradigm shifting daily until a difficult conversation Julie and I had over dinner one night. It began with a surprising, but fair, question: "Do you think you really have changed, or is it just because of your diagnosis?" I didn't know what to say. As my person, Julie is always pushing me and challenging me at all times. It is one of the many things I love about her, and she had every right to wonder. I had been a completely different person early in our marriage and even in the years leading up to that point in my life. I had been quick to anger, uncommunicative, and often inattentive. Now, I was trying to live a life completely devoid of all those traits. "Well, no, I don't want to be alone," I said. That made it much worse, but I couldn't understand why.

I woke the next morning in the guest room, and the first thing I thought about were the words I had said to her. Excitedly, I ran to our bedroom, woke Julie up, and said, "I figured it out!"

"Figured what out?" she said, sleepy and confused.

"Why you were upset last night. I heard the words. I told you that I don't want to be alone. What you heard is that I'm clinging to you because I'm *afraid* to be alone. What you don't understand is that I've always been alone. I believe I will always be alone. I'm fine being alone. But you make me not want to be alone."

That revelation opened a floodgate of thoughts on everything and everyone else in my life. That was why I wanted to open the foundation. That's why I fight so hard. That's why I am investing in a company focused on a culture of support. These are the people I want to be with, and I'm fighting tooth and nail for them. The foundation is really about the kids that I tend to gravitate toward: the ones who are living in neglect and clinging to hope for a better future, for love, for belonging.

The floodgate and the work I'm doing with our youth led me to answer another call, one that I had been trying to ignore for years. Still believing I would die at forty-five, I knew I needed to make peace with my childhood. To do that, I would need to have a deep and painfully honest conversation with my mother.

After calling to make sure it was fine for me to visit, I went to her house one afternoon and sat with her in her living room. We spoke about our shared past—our pain, our struggles, our regrets—and then we surrendered to each other. It wasn't easy, nor was it always perfect, by any means, but we ended our conversation agreeing to talk more so we could understand each other's experience with our past.

*

Through it all, I have come to see God's hand at work in the intricate tapestry of my existence. His plan, though often veiled in mystery, continues to unfold with each passing moment. It is a plan marked by twists and turns, by detours and dead ends, but through it all, I have learned to trust in the wisdom of His design.

It's difficult to say exactly why it took me so long to surrender to God's will for me. I had never been one to "tap out" easily, to submit to anyone or anything without putting my all into the fight. That mentality had made me a good wrestler and a good worker. I saw everything as a battle, a struggle in which I was an underdog and had to fight a little harder than everyone else to overcome. I had seen life through that lens for so long that I didn't know when it was good for me to surrender. The sheer act of it looked like failure to me, something to avoid at all costs. I suspect that I resisted the true consideration of anyone else's ideas or plans as they related to my own life because I felt that I would be surrendering my own ideas and plans to theirs, and how could theirs be better than mine? If they were superior, I was determined to make mine even better and carry on in my own headstrong way. I only knew how to push and grind forward. But when that mentality seemed to have led me to a dead end and seemingly with no one who wanted my company, I was forced to reconsider my ways.

I was implored by God to shed the person I had unwittingly, stubbornly allowed myself to become. My journey to this moment was a long and arduous one, paved with the sacrifices I had made in pursuit of professional success. I believed wholeheartedly that I had everything under control and could single-handedly pull down from the stars everything that my family and I would ever need or want. I felt invincible, unstoppable. It was my mission in life to prove this to be true. In reality, though, I was a workaholic. I was relentlessly chasing the next promotion, the next big deal. My wife and daughter became distant figures on the periphery of my life, overshadowed by the looming specter of the very ambitions that I believed would give them everything they ever wanted and needed. I never considered that maybe they only wanted *me*, in my full presence before them at the dinner table, at a school play, or during a family weekend. I consoled any doubts that arose within me by telling myself that I was providing for them all that I had ever wanted, oblivious to the toll my absence was taking on them.

I had never thought much about the passage of time until I found myself sitting in a sterile hospital, listening to those cold, clinical words: *multiple sclerosis*. Those two words echoed in my mind, drowning out everything else. Multiple sclerosis—a relentless thief, robbing me of control over my own body, my own life. At that moment, it felt like my world was crumbling around me, but little did I know that it was just beginning to rebuild.

As the diagnosis sank in, I found myself at a crossroads. My once-promising career came crashing down around me just as my symptoms worsened, leaving me feeling more isolated and unsure of my identity than ever. Suddenly, I was faced with a harsh reality: I had spent so much time building a life that was slipping through my fingers, so now what was I to do with what was left?

Amid my darkest hour, I found solace in prayer. I poured out my heart to God, knowing that I had not been my best self, much less a good believer, in years. I begged for guidance, for strength to face the uncertain road ahead. And slowly, almost imperceptibly, I began to feel a glimmer of hope. I had to let my old self die, to say goodbye to that version of me that had brought me here, in order to become the person I needed to be from here on.

As I delved deeper into my faith, I realized that true strength didn't come from worldly success or material possessions. It came from within, from the unwavering belief that I was loved unconditionally by a higher power. It was a revelation that shook me to my core, forcing me to confront the emptiness that had consumed me for the last several months after leaving work behind.

With each passing day, I felt myself shedding the layers of my old self—the zealous career man who had sacrificed everything for success, the numbness of my youth, the inattentive husband and father. In his place emerged a new version of me, one who was more thoughtful, sensitive, and introspective. It was a transformation that took both my family and me by surprise, as if I were rediscovering a part of myself that I had buried beneath the weight of my ambition.

But perhaps the most surprising revelation of all was the realization that the person I was becoming was not so different from the child I had once been—the neglected boy who had found safety and comfort in the arms of a loving God. In embracing my faith, I was rediscovering the innocence and purity that had been lost in the arduous pursuit of worldly gain.

After the launch of the foundation Beegins with You and Julie's decision to attend law school, we chose a trustworthy and reliable team to help us run the foundation. I was initially hesitant and unsure of the changes, the inexperience, and some of the ways to handle things, but I listened—truly listened—to everyone's point of view and finally understood the power of letting go of our own plans, which we are often convinced are the best and only way forward. For Julie and me, it felt like a moment in which both of our lives were finally aligning again, as if we'd come full circle.

One night over dinner, when Lucy was on the brink of turning twenty-one, Julie and I asked her how she wanted to celebrate her milestone. Her answer was one that I think every parent quietly hopes to hear: "With you." Before I knew it, Julie, Lucy, and I were driving on the highway toward Disneyworld, ecstatic and full of songs and our *Scooby-Dooby-Doo's* of anticipation. As we drove along the interstate, without warning, one of the car's tires went flat. I had always been the one who stepped in and took care of any kind of problem like this in the past. But in that moment, I knew I could not be that same person. However, I was stubborn and determined enough to try anyway. I spent hours trying to change the tire, with Julie periodically getting out to check on me and offering to assist. I did not like Julie helping me. Sitting idle on the side of a major highway with cars zooming by, it made me uncomfortable, but I know I could not have done it without her help. It took everything out of me, and what should have taken about half an hour took much longer, even with Julie's help.

We finally changed out the flat and were off to the airport to catch a later flight to Orlando. I was frustrated not to have been able to fix our predicament as quickly and easily as I once could, but I was still proud to have been able to resolve the problem and get my family to Disneyworld that night. I realized that the whole thing had just been me battling this entire situation. It turned out, though, that getting that flat tire was the best thing that happened to us, because it ruined every plan we had. Changing a tire is not a big deal, but that day it was. To be that tired and numb from such an insignificant ordeal was horrible, but it was also usefully humbling. It reset every expectation I had for myself, and it forced me to allow others to help me when I needed it.

We arrived at Disneyworld Wednesday night, giving us Thursday to explore the park before Lucy's birthday that Friday. The first place we went was Disney's Hollywood Studios. As we walked through the gate, Lucy said that she really wanted to ride one particular roller coaster. I volunteered myself as a co-passenger without hesitation. "Dad, you'll get sick," Lucy said. "I don't care about that. I can control it. I want to ride with you," I said, a smirk spreading across my face. "Fine," she said, laughing because she knew what was to come. I did, in fact, get sick. Medics came; some hydration was needed. But Lucy will always remember that the first roller coaster she ever rode on her twenty-first birthday trip, she rode it with me. That we can share that memory was totally worth it.

Julie and Lucy continued the day without me, converting the day into a magical mother–daughter experience. The following day, her actual birthday, would go down as one of the most relaxing days in history for us three as a family. Then Saturday, our last day of the trip, Julie stayed in the room to do her schoolwork. Lucy and I used that day for our father–daughter time.

The coaster incident really took a lot out of me, to the point that I required a wheelchair for the duration of Thursday and Friday. But when Lucy pushed a wheelchair up to me on Saturday, I shook my head. "There's no way I'm letting my daughter push me around in a wheelchair today." I opted to use Lucy for support when necessary and took plenty of sitting breaks, but we had a great day literally walking around the world at Epcot, exploring the beauty of the park, and connecting through deep conversation. It's one of my top memories of all time.

Our trip to Disneyworld reminded me of the importance of keeping moving. That no matter what—whether it's MS, the stresses of youth from not yet having enough answers to guide your choices, the inevitable pains of growing older, the indecisions that come along with both—you must keep moving. Keep trying. Stay curious and determined to progress to someplace better and to show others a way to get there once you find it. I keep moving simply by embracing my mistakes and discovering what I can learn from them. I accept my limitations, but I always look for ways around them, ways to supplant any skills or abilities that might have been diminished as time trudges onward, as it inevitably will forever and always. Let go of perfect, and you will find everything you need.

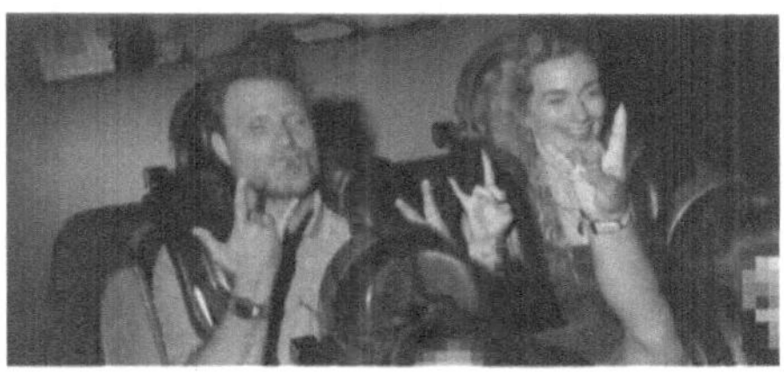

I was once pinned to a vinyl mat during a wrestling match at my school. I was sweating and heaving beneath my opponent, pondering how I would slip his hold and regain my control. I remember looking over to the sidelines and seeing Coach Chang, Digger, James, Mickey, Lisa, my dad, and a blurry row of classmates and townspeople. I could vaguely hear their desperate screams, cries, and, presumably, some instructions. But in the moment, I couldn't clearly make out any of their words. It was all just a wave of fervent screeching that I tried unsuccessfully to interpret as I lay on my back being ground into dust. I think often about that moment. I think about how I fought to remain calm. I think about Digger's, James's, and Coach Chang's faces; they looked like they would never have accepted my giving up, like there was no way I couldn't escape. They believed in my abilities. They had so much faith in me that I had no choice but to believe in myself as much as they did. Sometimes, you need people whom you respect and trust to remind you to believe in yourself. Those are the people who will tell you that you can defeat the impossible at the exact moment when you have lost all hope in yourself. That sort of thing is vital to your existence.

I had a strange sort of approach to being pinned beneath another body, someone who was trying as hard as he could to get me to submit. I never felt panicked or angry. Instead, I felt an uncommon sense of calm, like it was where I was most comfortable. I knew how to use my energy efficiently and how to get my opponent to waste his. I waited for his mistakes, for him to effectively tell me how to defeat him, to solve this problem that was literally on top of me. I was weirdly comfortable there, in the chaos. I understood it, and I knew how to navigate a way toward surviving it. I knew how to suffer the feeling of being alone and desperate for help.

I rarely lost a match, but whenever I did, I didn't remember who stopped me. I only remembered whom they stopped me in front of: Coach Chang, my dad, Mickey and Lisa, Digger and James. Each one of them never made me feel like anything but a winner, no matter what. They cheered for me whether I won or lost and always reminded me of everything I had done right, everything I would be able to do next time. But I always felt as though I had let them down and that I was less of the superhero I wanted to be for them, vowing to myself that I would never make the same mistakes again. In that way, those losses helped train me for life itself. I learned to remain calm under the weight of extreme pressure, to search for a solution even when my submission seemed imminent, to believe that I could outthink the unthinkable. In short, I learned not to give up.

As far as self-esteem and hopefulness were concerned after my diagnosis, though, I was at my lowest. Voices ruminated in my head, suggesting a thousand reasons why I should be angry and feel sorry for myself. Every one of them made some valid points. So much so that I could have remained stuck in anger and resentment and been forgiven for it. Then I began to hear a voice challenging me. "If all of that is true, then what? What will that mindset build, and where will it take you? *How will it make your life more enjoyable?*" As God's grace poured out upon me, He showed me how He has always been with me, working through those around me. Then I remembered Coach Chang, Digger, James, and Dan. I thought about Crystal, about my mother and my father. I thought about Julie and Lucy. I thought about everyone who had ever known me and believed in me. I thought about everyone who had ever fought harder than I was fighting now. I thought about everyone who had ever needed me, who had ever received my best effort, and then I heard that voice once again: "*If you were that person once, why can't you be that person again, My way?*"

My diagnosis was not the curse I had initially believed that it would be. Instead, it was a blessing that just took time to reveal itself. The ensuing unearthing of its gifts was a wake-up call that forced me to reevaluate my priorities and rediscover the true meaning of life. As I walk this new path now, I do so with a newfound sense of purpose and a deep faith that carries me through each day, even across the darkest ones that I must inescapably confront.

Throughout my life, I have seen God work through others for me. I now choose to allow Him to work through me for others because my new paradigm sees that God lives within everyone and only wants me to be in the present moment to witness His glory. I no longer need to imagine my future, and I'm left filled with a sense of gratitude. Although He is still teaching me, I am thankful for the lessons I have learned, the lives I may have touched, the love we have all shared through times that have at once and separately been easy, impossible, devastating, miraculous, and, in the end, life-altering. And though my own chapter may be ending, my story and that of our foundation is just beginning. May it serve as a testament of God's will for us to love one another and to the power of purpose, the resilience of faith, and the enduring legacy of hope.

In the end, perhaps the greatest legacy of all is to be used for God's glory and to strive for people to see Jesus living through us. In a world often shrouded in darkness, by simply living for others to see His presence, then we will serve as a beacon of light, illuminating the path for those to help others by loving others and daring to dream of a better way to live and always, always wrestle for the truth.

~

... it's about giving all the glory to God, our Father.

Our Father, who art in Heaven. Hallowed be Thy name. Thy kingdom come, Thy will be done in my heart, on Earth, just as it is in Heaven. Lord, I am grateful for everyone You have ever placed in my life, good or bad. I pray for Your blessings upon them all. I am grateful for Your will, Your knowledge, Your understanding, and Your wisdom. I pray to be Your vessel, Your servant, and part of Your eternal family. All things in my life are blessings from You; I choose to turn them back to praise for Your glory. Thank You for Your presence in my life. Thank You for guiding me through all things. Thank You for never allowing me to be alone. I love You. I ask all these things in Your son's name: Jesus, Yeshua, the Christ. Thank you, Father, for sending Your son to live as our blueprint and to die as our sacrifice, only to rise to be my savior. Now, may the words of my mouth and the meditation of my heart always be acceptable in Thy sight, My Lord, my strength, and my redeemer. Amen.

MY TWO CENTS

A REFERENCE FOR THOSE LIVING WITH MS

Receiving a diagnosis of MS is incredibly, incredibly hard. There's no doubt about that fact. It's natural to feel anger and frustration toward the world and everyone around you. Unfortunately, in my experience, holding on to this anger doesn't serve any purpose and will only make it impossible to move forward with your life, to gain anything better for yourself from this moment. Here are some insights and advice based on my personal experience of living with MS.

EMBRACE YOUR EMOTIONS, BUT KEEP MOVING

It's vital that you acknowledge the emotional impact of an MS diagnosis. Allow yourself moments to feel and vent, but don't let these emotions consume you. Remember, life only feels stagnant if you remain still. By continuously moving forward, you will convert challenges into opportunities to learn, grow, and strengthen. Ultimately, they can be very rewarding and enriching experiences in your life. Dive deep into understanding MS—its causes and potential treatments. You may uncover a strength within yourself you didn't know you had and realize that you're not alone in this. Many find solace and healing in their faith, recognizing that a higher power is there to provide guidance and support. I know I do.

Many of us get mad at the world when receiving a diagnosis such as MS, especially at a young age. I did. But again, being mad at the world just means that the world is winning. It won't accomplish anything for you. You cannot truly understand the "whys" of your life, nor can you fully appreciate its highs, its joys, if you allow anger and sadness to control how you view yourself and the world that you inhabit. However, I do understand the emotional experience, the trauma. You have to allow yourself a time and place to be emotional, to vent, and to be angry and scared, but do not allow yourself to forget that this struggle only gets worse if you stay there, if you stand still. If you keep moving, it's just another chance to gain strength, a new perspective, an opportunity to improve and help others. If you keep moving, you'll find out a lot more for yourself that can help you in this fight.

You might find out things such as the fact that MS has many causes or even go down rabbit holes to learn that it's a man-made disease. People even develop theories such as MS being a lazy diagnosis. In my own opinion, if you continue to look deep enough, you'll find strength, and you'll find that you are not alone. As I did, you may find that God is here, and He can provide healing.

The other two bits of advice I would offer are also just my opinions. These are things and experiences that I have gone through, and I in no way recommend anything that I have not tried myself. I'm only going to point out the things I believe have shown me great results.

The first topic is health. Below is a list of natural vitamins, minerals, and supplements that I include in my routine. You can do your own research to determine for yourself, but for me, there are common denominators here that help with many different health problems.

The other topic is about how I care for my mental and spiritual health. Again, these are just things that I have been doing over the years that have improved my quality of life, and hopefully they can help improve yours as well.

PRIORITIZE YOUR HEALTH

1. **Vitamin D3:** Check your levels and keep them elevated. Mine are low, so I use 10,000 international units daily.
2. **B12 injections:** 1–1.5 milligrams, twice a week. The older we get, the harder it becomes to absorb; using the liquid injection will ensure the body does absorb it.
3. **L-Lysine:** Two to three tablets daily. This is great for confusing viral loads, allowing your body to improve its ability to detox.
4. **Coconut chips** (as recommended): I do this periodically because coconut chips bind to viral loads in your bloodstream to help your body detox.
5. Listen to your body and **exercise**. Do so according to your limits, yet strive for a minimum of three times per week.
6. Try to eat **single-ingredient foods**. Stay away from preservatives and processed foods as much as possible.
7. **Drink plenty of water**. (Roughly half your body weight in ounces per day. Someone weighing a hundred and eighty

pounds, for instance, should drink about ninety ounces of water every day.)

8. Go **ninety days without sugar** and reintroduce at your own tolerance.
9. Get on a set of good **probiotics** (as they say, "gut health is your health").
10. For pain, stiffness, lethargy, or nausea, I use ten milligrams of **cannabis** as needed.
11. These are all things that I have done, and I love them.

SOME BONUS OPTIONS

A: A complete **tick-borne disease panel**. Use the company IGeneX, or a similar company, to verify all possible threats, such as Lyme disease, alpha-gal, and bartonella.

B: **Detox your body**. You can use foot pads or otherwise, but look for natural ways to detox your body daily.

C: Try an **eighty-four-hour fast**. Drink as much water as you can (at least half your body weight in ounces) per day. If you like, you may have one container of beef broth in the first and second twenty-four hours of the fast but thereafter water only. For more information, look online. It's a very common fast and invokes your body's healing system.

D: See an **acupuncturist**. It's more than needles! Many use holistic and natural methods to restore body function. It's been around for hundreds of years for a reason!

MEDICATION INSIGHTS

The last thing I will say about health is that, in the event you are taking medication recommended by your doctor, of the ones I have reviewed, I feel the most comfortable about **Copaxone**. It appears to be the oldest and safest and appears to pose the lowest amount of risk to your body. My understanding is that it adds materials to your bloodstream that protect your myelin from being attacked. It appears that any of the other medicines offered might suppress your immune system, a methodology I am very cautious about and not a fan of. I sincerely encourage you to always do your own research and be comfortable with the findings. Ultimately, it is your decision, so don't rush it, research it.

NURTURING MENTAL AND SPIRITUAL HEALTH

Taking care of your mental health is as important as your physical health. My faith has been a source of immense strength. For a long time, I felt alone, but through Scripture and prayer, I realized that I was never truly alone. Here are my suggestions for nurturing your faith:

- Read Scripture: Regularly engage with the Bible.
- Pray: Pray daily, not for yourself or material things but for others and for guidance.
- Gratitude: Cultivate a sense of gratitude. Be thankful for everything around you, which can bring new strength and even healing.

BONUS TIP: When you combine the nurturing of your mental/ spiritual health with tip "C" above, then you will be feeding yourself the bread of life!

If *faith* is a term of discouragement, or even if you don't know how to begin creating a regimen to deliberately practice obtaining your goals, then I would recommend looking into a program called the "I GOT This" framework. This is a tool to help you define who you are or want to become. This tool can help focus and transcend emotion into tangible control and goals within your life.

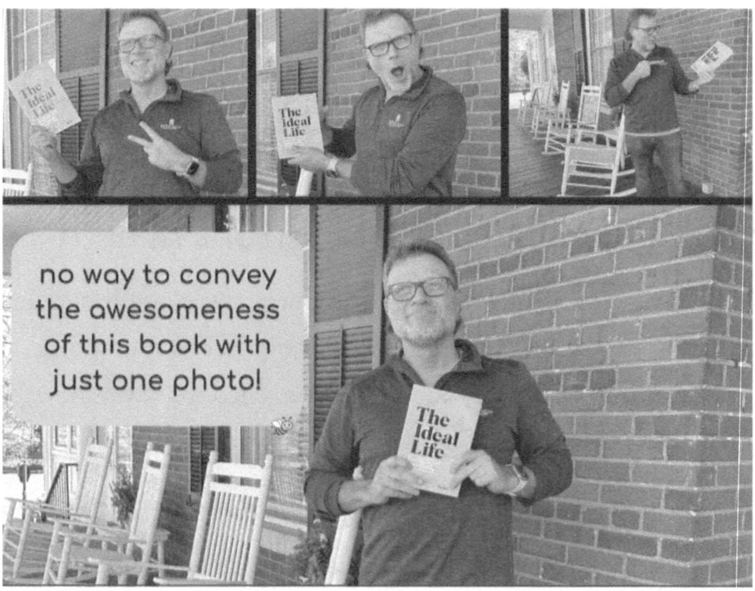
no way to convey
the awesomeness
of this book with
just one photo!
The Ideal Life

This program helped me slow down and reexamine my priorities one at a time. I like to call it the "order of operations for life!" Much like PEMDAS (parentheses, exponential, multiplication, division, addition, and subtraction, showing the priority order of operations from left to right) governs proper math, this framework provides a structure that helps you determine, design, develop, and deploy strategies to help you achieve your "Ideal Life"!

QUIET TIME AND MEDITATION

I cannot stress enough the importance of your mental health. I check in with my mental well-being through my faith. Personally, that's where I find a lot of the source of my strength. For the longest time, I felt that I was on my own, I was doing things, and I was moving straight ahead. And as I continue this path of learning and of not allowing the world to beat me or to win, I have learned that I was never alone. He was always within me, and I learned this through Scripture and prayer. I spent a lot of time in prayer, and my prayer life helped strengthen my mindset. But most of all, be grateful; be grateful for how God and the people in your life love you. Take notice of the special people around you and find gratitude for their help and love. Be grateful for everything around you that brings you joy and comfort. You will find new strength in that gratefulness. You will find new skills and a sense of peace and hope as well.

Outside of prayer, I like to spend a lot of time in meditation. In my quiet time, I like to listen to songs on repeat. I recommend listening to songs that inspire introspection. Here are some of my personal favorites:

1. "Nobody" by Casting Crowns
2. "Who You Say I Am" by Hillsong Worship
3. "Out of My Hands" by Jeremy Camp
4. "The Answer" by Jeremy Camp
5. "Blessed Be Your Name" by Matt Redman

6. "Awesome God" by Caleb + Kelsey
7. "Open the Eyes of My Heart" by Shane & Shane
8. "Blessed Be Your Name" by Tree63
9. "My Desire" by Jeremy Camp
10. "Thrive" by Casting Crowns
11. "My God Is Still the Same" by Sanctus Real
12. "The Comeback" by Danny Gokey
13. "One More Song for You" by Casting Crowns
14. "Keep Me in the Moment" by Jeremy Camp
15. "The Glory" by Kim Walker-Smith

All these songs are special to me. They are special, firstly, because of the words. But secondly, I listen to each song individually on repeat. As I do, it's not the song that I listen to—it's the introspective thought that this time creates. This is what works for me. This puts me into a state of thoughtful meditation. So, I highly encourage you to find something that allows you to enter into a calming state of gratitude, introspection, and contemplation at least once every single day. Something that makes you think about the things that you're going to be grateful for. The things that you were gifted by God. What are those talents you begin to realize? That is when you'll discover things about yourself that you have never found before.

For me personally, I also find reading Scriptures to be incredibly helpful and reassuring. Some of my favorites, in no particular order, are as follows:

- Galatians 5:16–18
- Job 28:28
- 1 Corinthians 8:2
- 1 Corinthians 16:14
- Proverbs 6:6–8
- Philippians 2:4
- Psalm 51:1–19
- Psalm 19:14
- Colossians 3:12–17
- Romans 5:3–5
- Ephesians 2:8–10
- Philippians 2:12–16
- Philippians 4:8–9
- 1 Chronicles 29:10–13 (David's Prayer)
- Hebrews 11:6
- Hebrews 12:4–12
- Romans 12:9–21
- John 16:13–15
- 1 Peter 3:8–22
- Ephesians 3:16–19
- Jeremiah 33:3

HELPING OTHERS

Helping others can be incredibly rewarding. It not only provides exercise but also fills your heart with love and purpose. When you help others, you often find that you receive just as much in return. You may even find healing, especially if you get out and help others. That's a great "two birds with one stone." You get your exercise, and by being out there and helping people, God gives you His dose of love, His dose of knowing you are there, His dose of using you and using others to help you. That's an amazing feeling and yet another thing to be grateful for. Facing MS is undeniably difficult, but with the right mindset and support, it is possible to find strength, hope, and healing. Embrace your emotions, prioritize your health, nurture your mental and spiritual well-being, and never hesitate to help others. These steps can transform your journey with MS into a path of resilience and discovery.

ACKNOWLEDGMENTS

The sharing of this story is not possible without the following people:

- Mark Congdon: I don't quite remember the year we began working together, but in the beginning, our paths only crossed as subject matter experts. However, once you began to work directly for me, we also began working more closely together. I was very impressed with your initiative, commitment to regiments, and market intelligence. So much, in fact, that I made it my personal mission to bring you out of the shadows so others could see your talents. As it would happen, you made another impression on me some years later by providing me with an opportunity to share my story and learn about the tools you used to impress me years earlier in our lives. This provided me with great insight, allowing me to learn the "why" behind your creation of the framework. Your trust to pull back the curtains of The Ideal Life opened yet another opportunity for God to minister to my heart. Your program not only forced me to slow down but also opened my mind to the scientific side of the God-given chemicals: dopamine, oxytocin, serotonin, and endorphins. Thank you for encouraging me to participate in both the program and with your wonderful staff. You have a great team, a great product, and a very powerful "why." May God bless you in all that you do, and know that you will always have my support. Also, I must thank you, brother. Writing this book was truly the most therapeutic thing I've done in my life! I am so grateful for you and the timing of our reconnection—even more for allowing God to work through you to impact my life!

- Matthew Godbey: Wow! That took longer than you expected, huh? You signed up to be my editor, hands, and organizer for this whole process. Bet you didn't know you would have to be a therapist, a psychiatrist, or even a project manager to keep me focused. All kidding aside, your skills are remarkable. Trust me, if I had done this alone, it would have been created using Excel. Thank you for helping me understand the logic behind the art of storytelling. Moreover, thank you for your patience with me. Memories and words are difficult to come by, yet this is why I exclaim that your skill is amazing and a true God-given talent. Our time together has forged a deep bond, and I pray nothing but the best for you in all your endeavors. P.S. Keep me on the short list for when the big one comes over the mountain! 10–4, and thank you my friend!

Those who make up my life:

- My Uncle Mike: I say, "Thank you, Jesus!"
- My Poppa Ralph: Thank you for always "working it out."
- Coach Spencer Chang: I am so grateful to have known you and to have had the privilege to wrestle under your tutelage. I am so looking forward to seeing you once again!

- Coach Taylor Edwards: I guess it was somewhere around 2021 when you and I reconnected, or at least thereabouts. It was on that lawn where we reminisced about your friend Dan Manson. It was on that day, some twenty-four years later, that you clarified that Dan's condition was muscular dystrophy. Relearning this was an absolute blessing and could not have happened at a better time in my life. Thank you for that, and thank you for always believing in me and pushing me to be better.
- To the peeps on the ninth floor of the Curry building and the best suitemates ever (Sembe, Paul, Doug, Andy, and Digs): Cheers to *007*, *Mario Kart*, and of course the honey bear bong. Those turned out to be some of the best memories. You all were my home.
- My brothers at ΔΤΧ: There are so many great memories, but here are my top three:

3. Civil War (North versus South keg race and the infamous Mike Brown fishhook after I stole the North's tap).

2. Jim Beam and the chants of "Two men enter; Blake will leave."

1. Golf parties at the Castle. Oh, those apple-pie shooters!

I can sincerely say with all my heart, TILOS.

- To Carol, Pat, Barbra, Arnie, and Shirley: Be honest … I terrified you on that forklift, didn't I? I had so much fun working with you guys. I always loved the balance of deadlines and having fun meeting them. Thank you for caring for me and Derrick on those nights we slept in the parking lot out of fear of being late. The safety of the environment you provided was amazing; thank you for allowing me to be creative and for your focus to get things done!

- To Tim, Posey, Daniel, David, Ernie, and Patsy: Thank you for creating an environment that allowed me to grow a foundation to stand on … and for some of the best bologna steaks and venison BBQ around!
- To Bobby and the entire team at Ridgeway Clocks: I cannot thank you enough for allowing this kid to poke around and annoyingly take his job seriously.
- To Andre: Thank you for taking a chance on me and giving me a rope to climb. You are truly an economic mastermind. I miss the early days driving you around. Any chance I could, I would listen and learn. I am not only thankful for the opportunity; I am also grateful to have learned so much from you. I wish nothing but the best for you and the boys!
- To Mr. Muscatello, Jeb Bassett, and of course the wonderful team of Joan and Phyllis: Got a minute! Thank you for taking me under your wing as I entered the international realm of supply chain. You provided an amazing paradigm of what customer service should be. Thank you for both your patience and your pressure. I guess there were times size sixty-four bold red font was needed. Seriously, between that top-down push and working daily with Meredith's absolute intolerance for imperfection, this was the best way for me to enter this industry! I am, and will always be, so grateful for you all!

- To Gene Winters: Thank you for your belief in me and your willingness to always be honest with me. You kept me on my toes, and I appreciated you so much for that.
- To Wayne Gaumer: While I was getting my first degree and breaking into the supply chain industry, you provided me with great mentorship. This would lead to advice and, ultimately, develop into a friendship that I have always valued. Thank you for your willingness to listen and provide guidance over the years!
- To Jimmy Foster: We have so many stories together, my friend. You have been a great and sporadic (Tigger-esque, even) part of my life. You were the very first person to tell me that I should write a book. Thank you for that encouragement and your friendship over the years. Having witnessed your complete career in the supply chain industry, I would have to define you as my GOAT salesperson. Everyone has their talents, yet I admire how you use yours for God's glory.
- To Neo: You are one of a kind. Thank you for your friendship, mentorship, and willingness to help me throughout the years. Your impression on me and my family will never be forgotten. I miss our lunches and honest conversations. You are a top-tier operator yet a higher-caliber man! Thank you again, my friend.
- To Lionel: We have seen some unbelievable things together. From being harassed for loitering at our own office space to hotdog heart attacks at hotels to varying stages of people-watching, we have experienced a lot together. We always seemed to be in the wrong places at the right times on the road together. Maybe one of the harder things to understand

is why our keyman policies made us more valuable dead than alive. Worse yet, it meant we could not travel together. Crazy times! I miss our friendship and how well we worked together. Thank you for being you.

- To Angela Haddox: You will forever be in my heart. William is so lucky to have you as his mother! Thank you for inspiring everyone you meet. You are one of those bright shining beacons of this world! Thank you, and I love you.
- To Bryan Beam: The year was 2012. You and I went to lunch at a local BBQ joint in Columbus, Ohio. It was that day, that car ride even, when I began to learn more about your amazing career. It wasn't until we hit a few snags in the rollout of the platform that more difficult conversations occurred and I began to be awestruck by you. Thank you for your ability to communicate with composure and, more importantly, your veracity to find the truth. I know I am just one of the many you have and continue to inspire. You are proof that the workforce is also a mission field and see everything as target-rich environments! Man, I love that! Thank you, brother!
- To Darren Brown: Thank you for your mentorship, your friendship, and how well we understood one another. It's my prayer that you have found your point of respite. Thank you for being such a great friend, but I rarely miss those all-nighters! You truly are among the smartest people I've worked with. Thank you for all you taught me.
- To Doug McBee: Although we did not have the opportunity to work together long, I want you to know I enjoyed our friendship, our talks about our savior Jesus Christ, and your

commitment to never compromising your faith. I know He has a great calling for you. Thank you, brother!

- To the individuals who I thought would be the future of the company (Jerry Fackler, Jon-Michael Norman, John Patterson, Bryan Schroeder, and Riggs Roberson): You all are among the most talented group of people I've worked with during my career. Granted, you each have a completely different skill set, yet you are each capable of doing anything you set your mind to. As we worked together, you each proved initiative and a myopic focus at your craft better than my own. I want you to know how proud I am of each of you. Thank you for your part in this journey to be a sponge and outperform! Most importantly, thank you for your friendship. We may not see each other often, but our bond was forged during a time of high pressure. That's supposed to mean it's strong, just in case my analogy is wrong, before you guys correct me—but then again, I've always loved our ability to be honest with one another! I will always be proud of each and every one of you!
- To Jessica Ingram: Many will ask, "What makes her so special?" I would first suggest that the correct question is, "Who made you so special?" Second, you and I know the details, but you are sincerely one of the most determined people I have ever met. Of the many, many people I have brought into my office and explained to as plainly as I could how to keep their job (which often requires a 180-degree change in behavior), you are the only person I have ever given that speech to and then seen make that turn. It has to be something that runs in your family. You are more than a fighter. You are aware of your surroundings and able to adapt. That's always been my

impression of you. Thank you for being an inspiration to me through your spirit to continually improve. Oh, that is such a powerful quality you have!

- To Vicky Steele: Wow, we have known each other a long time! So long, in fact, that you are like my great-grandmother of the supply chain! I know. I just made another age joke. This time, it's in writing … and others will see it! In all seriousness, we worked together at Pulaski, FIRSTCO, and the NEWCO, and then you retired at alliancebee. If I had to pick a mother of my supply chain career, it could only be you. I am so grateful to have known you and for you to have become such a positive influence in my life. I know you did this for others as well. Thank you. I love you and desire nothing but the best for you!
- To Rick Festa: We have worked together for a long time. You were the first person I hired back at FIRSTCO. And then when leaving FIRSTCO, you (unexpectedly) dropped a bombshell of an email. From there, you also became my first hire at the NEWCO. Thank you for your loyalty, friendship, and, most importantly, your love for Jesus and willingness to maintain that as your top priority. I so look forward to our coffee days! I'm so thankful you were with me for many parts of this journey.
- To Brad Ferguson and Lori Fox: I think when Michael Jordan was inducted into the Hall of Fame, he said something to the effect of "you never saw me without Pippen." I hope as you finish out your careers, you can remember me as your Pippen. You truly are the MJs of your field, yet, more importantly, you work with such honesty and compassion. I am so

grateful to have met you both; you are true forces of nature and will always have my willingness to support in endeavors of both life and business. Beyond that, you guys are some of my greatest and best friends! I love you both!

- To the rest of my NEWCO family: There is no way I am listing everyone, but I want to. I so very much loved working with each one of you. Whether your memories of our interactions are good or bad, I was simply trying to move you. The funny part is that, as I look back at our interactions and memories, it was all of you who were moving me. For that, I am eternally grateful. As a group, you truly accomplished amazing feats and, more importantly, created a culture where others wanted to be. Thank you so much. XOXO.
- To Eric: Despite the manner in which our relationship ended, I have come to realize you were a godsend to me. You were both a teacher and catalyst in my life. I earnestly could not have stepped out into a world of investment bankers and financiers without the opportunity to shadow and learn from you. I sincerely want you to know that I am grateful for our time together and wish nothing but the best for you and your family.
- To Angela Williams-Madiane: Although we met much later in my career, we spent a significant amount of time together talking and developing solutions for your teams. During our time working with one another, you focused on both of our teams and the culture we needed to be successful. I followed your lead and helped you create an environment where each of our teams developed into a little family. This was so much fun. I loved working with you and your team. Thank you for

your care and support when I needed you—especially for that time you drove me to urgent care. I am so grateful to have met you and to be part of the family you and Ryad create with all of those in your inner circle. I know our meeting was another beautiful blessing from God. I trust He has more lives in store for you to shine for His glory.

- To Mark Carlson: From the day we met, I have always been intrigued by your skills, stories, and level-headed approach to problem-solving. We were like peas and carrots talking through different solutions or options thereof. This was the beginning of a wonderful friendship. Trust began to set in as you helped open my mind through our personal discussions about personality types, etc. That's when I realized that we are not peas and carrots—you are simply the older version of me. I sincerely would love to be in your realm of experience and have the control of self you hold. You are truly one of the most skilled and accomplished people I know. You were an unlikely friend yet have become one of my closest. Thank you for your inspiration.
- To Jesse H. Wade III: It took over twenty years to answer the question, "Who are you for?" And Ben was right; he knew we would be friends if we actually spoke to one another. The timing of our reconnection and learning how wrong I was about who you are and how good of a person you truly are simply fanned a fire that God knew I needed lit within me. Thank you for being that catalyst to shift my paradigm. I am so grateful for our friendship.
- To my cohort from The Ideal Life (Karissa Tunis, Kate Slack, and our Coach Elizabeth Buckley): Thank you for your par-

ticipation in the I GOT This framework. The timing of our meeting on my journey was nothing short of another blessing turned lesson from God. You each impacted me dearly by simply equipping me with your strength, faith, and commitment to our goals. Thank you all for becoming my *Ideal Angels*; you slowed me down long enough to inspire me. I will always be so grateful for our meetings, and I look forward to each of our reunions and to learning how you affect and grow your circle of impact. Each of you is a wonderful beacon of light in this world!

- To Billy Boaz: Thank you for your unwavering focus on your path. You are an inspiration to me and to anyone who knows you. You have embraced the uncomfortable and are using it as a tool to learn, develop, and challenge yourself. This has and will continue to allow you to make a positive impact on the world. Many people get lost in the darkness, but through grace, time, and the help of many others, you were able to find your way. It's truly amazing what light can do in the darkest of times. It's been incredible to watch you on this journey. I pray that you embrace your light and know that your path has many great things in store for you. I'm so proud of you, and I want you to know that God loves you immensely. You will always have a fan in me. Believe that!
- To Brad Russell: We knew each other for nearly twenty years yet only became close friends during the last four or five. You were such a joy to work with, asking question after question. I called you my DIY customer. We rarely worked together on actual business transactions. However, if you wanted to know how to do something, I know I was one of the people

you would call—thus leading to you having the mentality of simply doing it yourself. It wasn't until our circles began to cross that our friendship blossomed outside of the workplace. This is where you would make the greatest impression on me. You lived your life lifting others up—from the kids on the teams you coached to the fans in the stands of the games you refereed or how you prioritized family and friends to ensure that you gave everyone some of your attention. You did so with genuine interest, concern, and intention to find the positive side of any situation. Thank you for living your life this way. Thank you for inspiring me and everyone you ever came in contact with to enjoy the blessing and love of one another during this life. Thank you for being one of the bright shining beacons in this world. Although you are no longer with us, the legacy of your life remains and will be a testimony I promise to keep alive! So, until we meet again, my friend, I praise the Lord for the time we had, and I trust you are now busy in eternity!

- To Jerry Lynwood Fackler Jr., a.k.a. J. L., a.k.a. "Worm": There are so many memories that come to mind when I think about you. There's how we met, a story of mistaken identity, or how you and I partnered up to dominate in cornhole tournaments, or the times when we teamed up to clean house at multiple company casino nights. While all of these memories are among my top ones, my favorite is the gift you gave me in your final days. You inspired a chat group, bringing together people who love the Lord and are willing to support one another through encouragement. Then, you and I were reunited through text messages, routine lunches, and open discussion about the Lord. Those conversations deepened when you started working at alliancebee. I am grateful for those conversations. I am so grateful to have known you and had the privilege to call you my friend. The truth is, you are someone that I will never be able to forget. I believe God interceded and brought us together, as He was also present with us through the moment we were separated by eternity. Thank you for giving me the greatest gift of all: the comfort to know I will see you again and we will continue to be a dominant team. All glory be to God!

My medical heroines and heroes:

- Dr. Janine Talty and Dr. Ben Thrower: Thank you for all you have done for me. I know our journey is not over, but I simply want to recognize that you both have a talent for listening. Your doing so—teaching me anew, or correcting my logic, or supporting me through challenges—has all impacted my life and helped me find my footing. I am so grateful for you both, and I can only believe that I was led to you through grace. See you soon!

My family:

- To Mom: I was in my forties when I found a copy of the 1979 class yearbook, for which you served as an editor, which included a picture of you bringing me to the school. This was the moment I realized I was in both the 1979 and 1997 senior annuals. Wow, how cool is that? I hope you know that I am grateful for everything you provided to ensure we had a home. At the time, I may not have understood, but I did know that you and Crystal needed me. I love you, and I am looking forward to getting to know that young girl who adored her baby boy.

- To Jim Easter: You grew to become one of my sister's favorite people. Thank you for being present and loving my sister. I know she loved you so very much, and that was enough for me. She was an incredible judge of character. Yet also, from my perspective, you are an extraordinarily kind man with a tremendous control of self. Thank you for your impact on my family's lives.
- To Mickey and Lisa: Thank you for taking me in and allowing me to have a front row seat to your family. The impact you have had on my life is profound—everything from Mickey pretending to be a tough guy to Lisa's ability to love so purely and unconditionally. I loved every moment of it, and I am eternally grateful for the experience and for your love for me as an unplanned extended family member. Love, your third son.
- To Teri: Thank you so much for being more than a stepmother. You have always been there, even when Dad could not be … oh, and thank you for not killing me when Dad wasn't around when I was grinding up the gears on the Mazda 6 back when you were patiently allowing me to drive your car. I love you so very much.
- To Dad: You once told me that people may not consider you a smart man, but you always try to surround yourself with smart people. That advice and how it helped me throughout my own career is proof that your wisdom transcends that of a man. I am eternally grateful for you and your love in every way. Moreover, thank you for being my greatest fan. In the

limited time we were together when I was growing up, you always used that time to focus on both Crystal and me. You are, and forever will be, one of my heroes. Thank you for always being present. I love you.

- To Joyce and Monroe Young: Our relationship has had its ups and downs. We never really got off on the right foot. How could we? Our worlds were colliding. The first several years that we knew each other, I lived in anger. I was so mad at the things I could not control. At the next collision, the unexpected occurred: Monroe confronted me. The most unexpected part was how he loved me. Thereafter, I worked harder. I watched as you and Joyce helped Julie raise Lucy while I was traveling or working late. Our journey has been far from easy. Through the grace of God, you continued to love me. You have no earthly idea the impact this has had on me. You have literally brushed the teeth of my soul with your love. Thank you so very much for that.

My brothers:

- To Robert Prillaman, Solomon Jappa, and everyone from the neighborhood: On a bike, we could do anything and go anywhere—graveyards, barns, tracks, ramps, creek chasing, fast getaways from places we were not supposed to be … and more. Andy from the TV show *The Office* hit the nail on the head when he said, "I wish there was a way to know that these are the good ole days when you are in the good ole days." From our trips to the arcade to *Bloodsport* kumites on the deck to pool parties, thank you for some wonderful memories that I may have not been so grateful for at the time. I miss you all.

- To Benjamin Smith: Whereas technically we grew up together, I would never say that. I would say that you defied who I thought you were when we reconnected at Longwood. From that day forward, I have looked at you like a little brother. After Julie and I were married, we called you our son. I know I am always hard on you. That is the reason why. Today, you continue to defy who people think you are, and that, my friend, is why I am so very proud of you! I will always love ya, bro!
- To Derrick Ingram: My brother from another mother! Watch out when you got that Diesel! Wow, the stories. The arguments. The struggles. Thank you for being a constant voice of truth in my life. I have seen you fight and lose to so many demons. Yet, you continue to fight on as if no one can put you down. It's been my honor to watch your career flourish as you create your own waves to surf. However, my greatest pride is seeing your faith in the Lord grow. You are a dangerous person, Derrick Ingram! Now get on the offense!
- To James Wells: Brother, I miss you so much. Anytime I think of you, I hear Digs yelling, "Slim!" There are so many memories of you exuding pure childlike joy. I have always said you were the rock of our group—not because you were literally unbreakable or would break anyone else but rather because of your intelligence, faith, and unwavering calmness in a storm. You truly were the best of us. One day, Digs and I will get our revenge on you as G.I. Joe's General Strike Base! One day, Joe … one day!
- To Digger Wells: When we met that day on the bus, something unusual occurred. It was like we entered a state

of quantum entanglement. No matter where we were or what we were doing, we were connected (at least that was my line of reasoning as to why we never lost playing spades). We have only seen each other a handful of times in recent years, but each time it is like we have always been together. I miss you, brother. You will always hold a special place in my heart. Although your and my paradigms of your family are different, I sincerely thank you for sharing and making me part of yours. I am so proud of the family man and successful entrepreneur you turned out to be. I will always be here for you. I love you, brother!

My sister:

- To Crystal: When we were little, you were my safe place and the person whose bed I went to when I was afraid. I love you, and I am sorry for leaving you alone. I know that you forgive me because I know that you knew someone I did not. I know because I, like you, can see Him working in the tapestry of my life now too. That was always your big secret. You knew you were never really alone. Thank you for everything you gave me; I carry and wear it daily. Love, Eyeee.

My world:

- To Chance: You were my first form of therapy. I never understood why you were taken from me so early. Yet, now I see that you completed your mission. I cannot wait to see you again!
- To my Lucy-Goose: Oh, how I love you so very much. You are a true gift of light to this world. Your capacity to love, work with others, and creatively design art or activities are true blessings from God. Your talent to connect with children is

uncanny. I pray for God's love to surround you and that you find joy in using your talent to serve His will. Never lose focus. Remember that we do not fight forces of this world, and that is why the battlefield is in our mind. I am so proud of you, and I know that He has so much in store for you. I love you and cannot wait to see you write the chapters of your life!

- To Julie: You are the Ironman of the story of my heart. There is no family without your love, without your ability to push through an adverse home life with me. I am so thankful for your prayers, for your love, and for your willingness to forgive me. I was horrible at creating a loving environment. Thank you for creating one for Lucy. Thank you for being her beacon of light when I would not be. Lucy is the greatest thing in this world, and I know I had little to do with that. Our marriage is something I believe could only be designed by God. As you built this environment, you pursued a career of talents. Now, as if by design, I shift more into the background to support you as you pursue your passions. Your love and determination know no bounds. You are the one and only constant of my life, and I am so thankful that He brought us together. You will always have my heart. I love you with all that I am—Captain Strange.

To the unknown:

- To all board members, investors, employees, and members of alliancebee: Your journey thus far has been so inspiring to watch. Your talent and dedication to your craft are amazing. Your story is truly one of my favorite things to witness. There has been no turn where God has not been present, and I am so grateful for the culture being created to embrace His love and will! Thank you all for your willingness to challenge the status quo and bring integrity to an industry that needs it; that is your true measurement of success!

- To all board members, students, and partners at Beegins with You, thank you for joining us on this journey. Thank you for the understanding that what we are doing as a group is bigger than our own ambitions. Thank you for the understanding that change begins in our own hearts and that we can help others by simply loving and supporting them, like the blueprint God gave us by sending His Son to love and forgive those He encountered. Thank you for your commitment to becoming the change we need!

To the known:

- Lastly, I know that I cannot receive forgiveness without first learning how to forgive. Therefore, I want everyone who has impacted my life, whether in this book, listed here or not, to know that I am grateful for each and every person in my life, both past and current. I carry some piece of you in my mind and heart. It is my prayer that there is a grand family reunion for us all, just maybe not in this world. Until then, I leave you with the words of Paul from 1 Corinthians 16:14: "Let all you do, be done in Love."

CONTACT US

Want to stop talking about problems with the youth and get involved with solutions for them instead? Check out more about our foundation. Get involved, donate, or start a new chapter in your community.

We are dedicated to becoming hands that help, ears that listen, feet that go, people who love, and hearts that begin change. Our goal is to make a positive impact on our community through environmental stewardship, educational enrichment, and social support. If you have any questions, need more information, or would like to get involved, please feel free to reach out to us through the following contact details:

Beegins with You Foundation

Mailing Address:
P.O. Box 4283
Martinsville, VA 24115
Phone:
Main Office: (833) 423-3446
Email:
General Inquiries: admin@beeginswithyou.org

Volunteer Opportunities: volunteer@beeginswithyou.org
Supporter Bee Program: supporterbee@beeginswithyou.org

Website:

www.beeginswithyou.org

Social Media:

Follow us on social media for the latest updates and news:

- Facebook: facebook.com/beeginswithyou
- Twitter: twitter.com/beeginswithyou
- Instagram: instagram.com/beeginswithyou

www.ingramcontent.com/pod-product-compliance
Lightning Source LLC
LaVergne TN
LVHW091548040926
847245LV00001B/8
* 9 7 8 1 6 4 2 2 5 9 0 7 0 *